Patterns of Nursing Theories in Practice

Patterns of Nursing Theories in Practice

Edited by Marilyn E. Parker

National League for Nursing Press · New York
Pub. No. 15-2548

Copyright © 1993
National League for Nursing Press
350 Hudson Street, New York, NY 10014

ISBN 0-88737-600-2

Library of Congress Cataloging-in-Publication Data

Patterns of nursing theories in practice / Marilyn E. Parker, editor.
    p. cm.
  Pub. no. 15-2548.
  Includes bibliographical references.
  ISBN 0-88737-600-2
  1. Nursing—Philosophy.
  [DNLM: 1. Nursing Theory. 2. Parker, Marilyn E.   WY 86 P316
1993]
RT84.5.P39 1993
610.73'01—dc20
DNLM/DLC
for Library of Congress   93-3402
                                            CIP

This book was set in Goudy and Caledonia by Eastern Composition, Inc. The editor and designer was Nancy Jeffries. Northeastern Press was the printer and binder. The cover was designed by Lauren Stevens.

Printed in the United States of America

*This book is dedicated to the nurses of South Florida
who have recently reminded us that in nursing
heroism is ordinary,
and to nurses elsewhere who responded
with courage and compassion
following Hurricane Andrew.*

Contents

Contributors

Charlotte Barry, BHS, RN
MSN Candidate
College of Nursing
Florida Atlantic University
Boca Raton, Florida

Anne Boykin, PhD, RN
Dean, College of Nursing
Florida Atlantic University
Boca Raton, Florida

Howard Karl Butcher, MScN, RN,
    PhD Candidate
College of Nursing
University of South Carolina
Columbia, South Carolina
Assistant Professor
School of Nursing
Pacific Lutheran University
Tacoma, Washington

Carolyn Padovano Corliss, MS, RN
Doctoral Student
Boston College
Chestnut Hill, Massachusetts

W. Richard Cowling, III, PhD, RN
Associate Professor of Nursing
University of South Carolina
Columbia, South Carolina

Anayis K. Derdiarian, MPH, DNSc,
    RN
Director, Nursing Research and
    Quality Improvement
Professor, School of Nursing
LAC + USC Medical Center
Los Angeles, California

Kathryn A. Edmunds, BN, RN,
Master's Candidate, Wayne State
    University
Community Public Health Nurse
Windsor-Essex County Health Unit
Windsor, Ontario, Canada

Keville Frederickson, EdD, RN,
    FAAN
Professor of Nursing
Lehman College, City University of
    New York
Clinical Nurse Scientist
Montefiore Medical Center
Bronx, New York

Carol Kearney, MSN, RNC
Boca Raton Community Hospital
Boca Raton, Florida

Susan Kleiman, MS, RN, PhD
    Candidate
Certified Clinical Specialist
Adult Psychiatric and Mental Health
    Nursing
Centerport, New York

Patricia Blanchette Kronk, BSN, RN
Clinical Supervisor, Community
    Home Health
Broward County, Florida

Madeleine Leininger, CTN, PhD,
    LHD, PhDNsc, DS, RN, FAAN
Professor of Nursing and
    Anthropology
College of Nursing and Liberal Arts
Director of Transcultural Nursing
    and Human Care Program
Wayne State University
Detroit, Michigan

Katherine McLaughlin, BScN,
    MScN, RN
President, McLaughlin Associates
MCL Educational Services, Inc.
Saskatoon, Saskatchewan, Canada

Gail J. Mitchell, PhD, RN
Nurse Scientist, The Queen
    Elizabeth Hospital
Assistant Professor, University of
    Toronto
Toronto, Ontario, Canada

Marilyn E. Parker, PhD, RN
Associate Professor of Nursing
Florida Atlantic University
Boca Raton, Florida

Rosemarie Rizzo Parse, PhD, RN,
    FAAN
Professor and Coordinator, Center
    for Nursing Research
Hunter College of The City
    University of New York
New York, New York
Editor, *Nursing Science Quarterly*
President, Discovery International,
    Inc.

Sister Callista Roy, PhD, RN,
    FAAN
Professor of Nursing
Boston College
Chestnut Hill, Massachusetts
Research Professor in Nursing
Mount St. Mary's College
Los Angeles, California

Savina O. Schoenhofer, PhD, RN
Associate Professor of Nursing
Graduate Progam Director
Florida Atlantic University
Boca Raton, Florida

Carole Schroeder, PhD, RN
Research Coordinator
Denver Nursing Project in Human
    Caring
Senior Instructor
School of Nursing
University of Colorado Health
    Sciences Center
Denver, Colorado

Dale M. Walker, BSN, MSc, RN
Executive Officer, Nursing
Vancouver Health Department
Vancouver, British Columbia,
    Canada

Cathie L. Wallace, MSN, RN
Adjunct Instructor of Nursing
Florida Atlantic University
Boca Raton, Florida

Vicki Yeager, RN
Staff Nurse, Adolescent and Child
    Psychiatry
Charter Hospital
West Palm Beach, Florida

Preface

This book and its companion, *Nursing Theories in Practice* (Parker, 1990) feature the major nursing theories of our time and highlight use of these theories in nursing practice. Each chapter is original work prepared by nursing theorists and nurses expert in study and use of nursing theories in the practice arena. All of the chapters written by nursing theorists are followed by one or more chapters written by nurses who use the specific nursing theory in their practice. Chapters offer clear evidence of connections of nursing theory and practice and support continuing development of nursing as a discipline of knowledge and professional practice.

This volume includes the most recent explication of the Roy Adaptation Model, Parse's Human Becoming Theory and the Culture Care Theory of Leininger. An emerging general theory of nursing, Nursing as Caring, is presented by Savina O. Schoenhofer and Anne Boykin. Josephine Paterson and Loretta Zderad have responded to continuing enthusiasm for their work by supporting Susan Kleiman in her chapters for this book on Humanistic Nursing Theory. The nursing theories and frameworks of Dorothea Orem, Dorothy Johnson, Jean Watson, and Martha Rogers that appear in the 1990 book receive continuing attention in this volume as nurses offer new information about the importance of each of these theories to their practice.

The title of this book invites consideration of the concept of pattern and the use of this concept to advance thinking about nursing theories and nursing practice. A pattern may be thought of as a form or design for making something. We use the word to describe taking action to make something according to a plan. Nursing theories may be thought of as patterns, as models to guide the making and doing of nursing. Nursing theories both reflect our thinking about nursing and offer ways to think anew about our practice. Nurses may bring data from their practice to the light of nursing theories and may refine or create nursing theories according to new understanding. Many nurses can expect the exciting realization that the essence of a nursing theory is consistent with their current practice; the pattern is being followed without full knowing. Our commitment and compassion for nursing is refreshed by our hopes for fruitful study and use of nursing theories.

Nursing as a body of knowledge and service to society needs theories. At the same time, nurses long for improved ways to understand and communicate about their practice. Nurses are willing and able to explore and inquire to make sense of the world of nursing and to make nursing practice better for their clients and themselves. Howard Butcher in Chapter 13 asserts that developing and using nursing theories in practice may be the most crucial task facing nursing today. Walker in Chapter 18 warns that great conviction and courage are required for exploring nursing theories to guide practice. So, we are advised that we must develop, study and use nursing theories as patterns for practice. And we are reminded to strengthen our commitment to nursing as we enter the venture of doing what must be done.

Both Rogers (1990) and Levine (1990) assure us that coordinated sense must be made of the empirical data of our world and that this can be done more fully in the light of nursing theory. The promise of this assertion and the notion of pattern are reflected in the format and content of this book and in its companion *Nursing Theories in Practice* (1990). Nursing patterns, our nursing theories, encourage dreaming and wondering, demand thinking and inquiry and invite the visions, solutions and new questions that result.

Marilyn E. Parker, PhD, RN
Boca Raton, Florida
January 1993

References

Parker, M. E. (Ed.) (1990). *Nursing theories in practice.* New York: National League for Nursing Press.

Rogers, M. E. (1990). Space-age paradigm for new frontiers in nursing, in M. Parker (Ed.). *Nursing theories in practice.* New York: National League for Nursing Press.

Levine, M. E. (1990). Conservation and integrity, in M. Parker (Ed.). *Nursing theories in practice.* New York: National League for Nursing Press.

Acknowledgments

The South Florida Nursing Theorist Conferences have provided a model of unity among nurses joined by love of nursing, respect for nurses as persons and professional colleagues, and commitment to greater understanding of nursing as a body of knowledge and professional practice. The forum has been structured in a manner which encouraged nurses to participate in open dialogue about nursing theory and nursing practice. Through this dialogue nurses have awakened opportunities to truly listen to each other and to know that without each other, those at the podium and in the audience alike, we cannot develop our nursing to its fullest. Indeed we must join, and listen and hear in order to know the richness of our community and come to share our thinking, longing, searching and our joy.

Most of the contributing authors of this book have been featured speakers at the 1991 or 1992 South Florida Nursing Theorist Conferences and have prepared original work for this book. One chapter anticipated for this work does not appear due to the death of the author, David B. Stasiak. His presentation at the 1991 Conference was much appreciated for clinical scholarship and challenging insights into use of Leininger's Theory of Culture Care.

Encouragement and help in preparing this book have come from many professional and personal sources. I have appreciated working with Sally J. Barhydt and Nancy Jeffries of the National League for Nursing who have consistently offered genuine interest, ability, and the cooperation necessary to produce such work. I am grateful to each one of the authors who contributed to this book and am honored to know them as friends and colleagues in our shared commitment to nursing. Gratitude is also due the many nurses who join this group as fellow participants in the study of nursing theories and nursing practice.

Part I

Introduction

1

Studying Nursing Theories for Use in Practice

Marilyn E. Parker

This chapter will explore some issues about using nursing theory in nursing practice and offer direction for studying nursing theories. Ideas for this chapter were stimulated by the South Florida Nursing Theorist Conferences and reflect dialogue with nurses in many service and classroom settings. Participants at the Conferences, like nurses in classroom and service settings, had varying education and practice backgrounds as well as diverse knowledge about nursing theory.

Questions that will be addressed are: What are key issues about using nursing theory in practice? What do I want from nursing theories to help my practice? Which nursing theories shall I study? How shall I study nursing theories for use in practice? Readers are invited to join nurses who contributed to development of this chapter by noting their own unique questions as well as many questions and viewpoints about study and use of nursing theory that have been shared among nurses.

ISSUES ABOUT USING NURSING THEORY IN PRACTICE

The overriding issue is how can nursing theory and nursing practice be brought together? This question recognizes that separation of nursing theory and nursing practice is artificial and that nurses can no longer

continue to see these two essential nursing endeavors in distinct settings, being the concern of either scholars or practitioners. Many chapters of this book and the companion volume, *Nursing Theories in
Practice* (Parker, 1990) offer direction for this issue. In fact, many
nurses find the values which guide day-to-day living also guide their
practice. These nurses realize that the values and assumptions which
form the basis for particular nursing theories are consistent with beliefs
that guide life. These nurses readily experience the joining of nursing
theory and nursing practice.

One exchange between a practicing nurse and a nurse theorist highlights the issue. A nurse speaking from the perspective of her own experience said: "What is the meaning of this theory to my practice? I'm in
the real world! I want to connect—how can connections be made between your ideas and my reality?" The nurse theorist responded with an
explanation about the values and assumptions of her theory. The nurse
in practice responded: "Yes, I know what you are talking about. I just
didn't know I knew it and I need help to use it in my practice."

The practice of nursing is lived moment-to-moment, day-to-day and
is guided by values, beliefs and knowledge held by the individual and by
groups of nurses. These values and beliefs ground nursing theories as
well as nursing practice. If nursing theory is practical, how can it be
useful in practice? What goals does it serve and how do these purposes
come into being? Can nursing theory help nurses to see beyond the
immediate facts of technology and learn to use demands of the care
system to access patients and provide avenues for nursing? Nursing theory must guide responses of nurses to both critical and ordinary nursing
questions.

We continue to assert that theory enriches practice and this is confirmed throughout this volume. Study and critique of both content and
processes of nursing theory are increasingly common in undergraduate
as well as graduate nursing education programs. Where are the nursing
practice settings that encourage further development and use of the
knowledge about nursing theory in the practice arena? Concerns of many
nurses include discontent that nursing theory evaluation and support for
application of theories is not present in practice. Therefore, the valuing
of that nursing theory in nursing practice is called into question.

We also assert that practice enriches theory. Consider the nurse
caring for the patient, or the nursing manager with a concern to facilitate nursing for patients in a setting. What are these nurses thinking

about? If the thoughts of these nurses are of nursing, the ideas must be connected to the content and structure of the discipline of nursing and therefore to nursing theory. Is it naive to propose that nursing theory development often takes place at the bedside and that nursing theories are refined daily in a variety of practice settings? Does unique and innovative nursing practice actually result directly from ongoing development and use of nursing theory by real nurses in real nursing situations? Why would development, analysis, and evaluation of nursing theory be so widely featured in nursing curricula if the expectation were not that nurses would use this content to direct and improve the day-to-day practice of nursing?

These and many other questions and issues belong to nursing and will be dealt with by nurses in practice, education, theory development, and research. Nursing theory must be used to help understand nursing practice. Nursing practice must contribute to ongoing developing nursing theory.

WHAT DO I WANT FROM NURSING THEORIES?

The major purpose of studying nursing theories is to advance the discipline and practice of nursing. More immediate reasons for studying nursing theory have been offered by nurses and are summarized below as questions. Many of these reasons may also be used as guideposts for developing and examining nursing theory. Several of the questions illuminate possible obstacles to use of theory.

- Is this a good theory according to opinions of knowledgeable and trustworthy nurses?

- Can the theory be understood in relation to nursing as I know it to be? Is it a real nursing theory for real nursing practice? Will it support what I believe is good nursing?

- Will I be stimulated without being overwhelmed? My mind needs this but can this really be useful outside the classroom?

- Are the terms usable? Do they encourage use and translation to others? Is the theory "user friendly"?

- Is the theory applicable to multiple clinical situations?

- Is there evidence that use of the theory may lead to markedly improved nursing care?

- Does the theory fit the subject matter of nursing?

- Does it lead to nursing research questions and methods?

- Has it grown and become richer over time?

- Will use of the theory be compatible with expectations of patients, other nurses, physicians and administrators so that conflict can be at a minimum?

- What is required for thinking about nursing theories in practice? What must I do? Am I able?

WHAT NURSING THEORIES SHALL I STUDY?

Nurses in practice, as individuals and as groups of nurses working together, wonder where to begin their study of nursing theory. This is also the first question asked by nurses in service divisions of hospitals and other care settings as consideration is given to selecting a nursing theory as a basis for administration and organization of nursing services. The following exercise is suggested as a first step in considering answers to this query. The exercise will clarify aspects of nursing practice for each nurse and from this information the nurse may provide data for decisions about further study of one or more nursing theories.

The exercise is based on the belief that study, selection, and use of nursing theory in practice must be grounded in the practice of the nurses involved and must reflect essential elements of that practice. Nursing theory and nursing practice are joined in nursing situations and it is from these situations that decisions about practice are made and come into being.

1. Select a quiet and comfortable place where you are unlikely to be disturbed. Reflect on your individual nursing practice and the enduring beliefs and values that brought you to nursing and that keep you in practice. What are the beliefs and values you hold most dear about nursing practice? From this reflection select a nursing situation that seems to best exemplify your practice and illustrates your nursing beliefs and values.

2. Describe the nursing situation. Who was the patient or client in the nursing situation? For example, who was he or she as a person? What were the needs for nursing of the person? What nursing responses did you offer to help with these needs? What other nursing responses might you have made? What was the setting of the nursing situation? What aspects of the environment were important to the need for nursing and what environmental factors influenced the nursing response?

3. Make notes about your process of reflection and write about your description of the nursing situation. You may choose to make these the initial entries in a journal recording your study of nursing theories in practice. Such a journal can be a way to observe your growth in study of nursing theories for use in practice. It can be a source of nursing questions for further study.

4. It is often in the reflecting, writing, and discussing of values and essential components of nursing situations that nurses come to fuller awareness and appreciation of their nursing. You may offer aspects of your process and of your nursing situation in discussion with nurse colleagues who are also seeking to select nursing theories for study. Sharing these experiences will serve to clarify your views and encourage support of not only the reflective process but of the nursing values and their illustration in the various nursing situations.

5. If you are in a group of nurses seeking to study nursing theories, it will be useful to share commonly held nursing values and beliefs as well as exemplars of nursing situations that represent practice of the group.

6. Use these values, beliefs, and nursing situations to help in choosing which nursing theories to study and consider for guiding practice. What nursing theories seem consistent with the identified values, beliefs, and nursing situations? Continuing reflection and writing in your journal will be major contributions to making your choices. What questions are important to ask? What do you want from use of nursing theory?

7. Use your questions to begin a literature search. Gather and use library resources. You may seek consultation for analysis or evaluation of specific nursing theories. Talk about the pro-

cesses of examining nursing theories and their use. This is a
time for exploring, learning and sharing, not for actually evaluating and judging. Enjoy your new insights and record your
questions as you continue to relax and learn. This process
should be stimulating, challenging, gratifying and often fun.

HOW SHALL I STUDY NURSING THEORIES FOR USE IN PRACTICE?

The study of nursing theories is empowering and dynamic. Nurses who
are intimately involved in nursing practice day-to-day are seeking their
places in the work of advancing nursing knowledge through examination of nursing theory. Discussions with nurses indicate the need for
criteria to evaluate nursing theory that hold particular meaning for the
nurse. Nurses ask for ways to know the *nursing* in the theory and to
appraise the nursing theory in light of their concerns with practice.
This is a call to go beyond evaluation of theory as theory although
evaluation of desirable attributes of any good theory in any discipline
must not be overlooked.

Using the Literature to Study Nursing Theories

Various guides for development, analysis, and evaluation of nursing
theories are available in excellent nursing texts; two of these are Chinn
& Jacobs (1991) and Fawcett (1984). Moody (1990) provides a thorough review of analysis and evaluation of nursing theory with a particular focus on nursing research. Several nursing theorists offer descriptions
of processes of development of their specific theories. Orem (1991),
Parse (1987), and Watson (1988) are examples. The current periodic
literature is rich with issues about theoretical development in nursing
and Nicoll (1991) contains papers from more than three decades of
theory development in nursing.

Studying Nursing Theories with a Focus on Practice

The following questions have been developed to facilitate study of nursing theories for use in nursing practice. This guide is intended to focus
on clear conceptions of nursing as well as points of interest and general
information about each theory. Each of the four major questions is sup-

ported by other questions that will enrich inquiry and understanding. Most of the questions may be used to study most of the nursing theories; other questions will be more useful when studying groups of theories, such as nursing theories created for a particular type of nursing practice. The questions are also useful for developing a survey of nursing theories.

This guide was designed for use by practicing nurses as well as by students in undergraduate and graduate programs of nursing education. Work by the Nursing Development Conference Group (1979) was an early stimulus for this guide and the questions are ever changing. Many practicing nurses and students have used these questions and contributed to their development.

Responses for these questions may be found in nursing literature and audiovisual resources in hospital and university libraries as well as in some textbooks and journals in personal libraries. It is important to use primary sources written by the nursing theorist or nurses who are recognized authorities in use of the nursing theory. Chapters in this book and in *Nursing Theories in Practice* (Parker, 1990) are ready resources for this study. Care should be taken to examine each question carefully; additional questions may be needed for particular purposes of inquiry.

The first major question will help define the nursing theory and illustrate use of the theory in nursing practice. Essential elements of the theory of nursing will be identified by working with the first major question. The second, third, and fourth major questions encourage curiosity about nurses in other times and other places and support connections among nurses in various avenues of nursing practice. These questions require further depth of study and invite a summary of information acquired in the overall inquiry.

A GUIDE FOR STUDY OF NURSING THEORIES FOR USE IN PRACTICE

1. What is the conception of nursing stated in the theory?

    • What is the focus of nursing? What does the nurse think about when thinking about nursing? What does the nurse give attention to? What guides nursing observations and decisions?

    • What is the purpose of nursing? What does nursing intend to accomplish? Why do nurses do what they do as nurses? How may quality and amount of nursing be described?

- How is nursing distinguished from other helping services? How is nursing related to other helping services? What are the limits of nursing set forth by the theory?

- In what situations is nursing practiced? What are characteristics of the nurse? What are attributes of the patient or client? What are the environmental requirements that set boundaries for the practice of nursing?

- What are illustrations of the use of the nursing theory to guide nursing practice? Is the richness and complexity of nursing practice evident in the use of the nursing theory? Cite scholarly literature, professional presentations, and experiences reported by knowledgeable colleagues.

2.   What is the context of development of the theory?

- Who is the nursing theorist as a person and as a nurse? Why did the theorist develop the theory? What are some of the central values and beliefs of the theorist? What does the theorist believe about the nature of being human?

- What nursing theories influenced the development of this theory? What nursing theories were developed before and concurrent with this theory? What nursing-related theories influenced the development of this theory?

- What were the major social, economic, and political influences of the time? What were images of nurses and nursing when the theory was developed? What was the status of nursing as a discipline of knowledge and profession?

3.   Who are authoritative sources for information about development, evaluation, and use of this theory?

- Who are recognized nursing authorities who speak, write about, and use this theory of nursing? What are professional and personal characteristics of these persons? What are attributes of authorities? How does one become an authority of the nursing theory? What other nurses should be considered authorities?

- What major books and articles describe the development, evaluation, and use of the nursing theory? What associations of nurses have been organized to support development and use of the theory? What nursing service and academic programs are recognized as main sources of information about the nursing theory?

4.   How can the overall importance of the nursing theory to nursing practice, scholarship, and education be described?

- What is the significance of the theory of nursing over time? To what extent has the theory been used to structure and guide individual and institutional nursing practice? Is the theory used to organize nursing knowledge in nursing education programs? Does literature include reports of research guided by the theory of nursing? What is evidence of ongoing development and evaluation of the theory?

- What is the experience of nurses who report consistent use of the theory to guide practice? Is nursing research guided by the theory of nursing regularly reported in the nursing literature? Has the theory led to development and use of methods of nursing inquiry?

- What are recognized as the key influences of the theory on the continuing development of nursing as a discipline of knowledge and professional practice? What are future possibilities for nursing and nurses based on this theory of nursing?

In the spirit of continuing the dialogue nurses are invited to participate in the ongoing work of forging connections of nursing theories and nursing practice. Nurses are invited to respond to aspects of this chapter with questions about using nursing theories in practice and ways to support effective study of nursing theories for use in practice. These responses will contribute to advancing nursing practice and move our discipline forward.

REFERENCES

Chinn, P., & Jacobs, M. (1991). *Theory and nursing: A systematic approach.* (2nd ed.) St. Louis: C. V. Mosby.

Fawcett, J. (1984). *Analysis and evaluation of conceptual models of nursing.* Philadelphia: F. A. Davis.

Moody, L. E. (1990). *Advancing nursing science through research.* Newbury Park, CA: Sage Publications, Inc.

Nicoll, L. H. (Ed.). (1991). *Perspectives on nursing theory.* Boston: Little, Brown and Co.

Orem, D. E. (Ed.) (1979). *Concept formalization in nursing: Process and product.* Boston: Little, Brown and Co.

Orem, D. E. (1991). *Nursing: Concepts of practice.* (4th ed.) St. Louis: C. V. Mosby.

Parker, M. E. (Ed.) (1990). *Nursing theories in practice.* New York: National League for Nursing Press.

Parse, R. (1987). *Nursing science: Major paradigms, theories and critiques.* Philadelphia: W. B. Saunders Co.

Watson, J. (1988). *Nursing: Human science and human care.* New York: National League for Nursing Press.

Part II

Humanistic Nursing Theory

2

Reflections On Knowing Josephine Paterson and Loretta Zderad

Susan Kleiman

While struggling with these chapters on Humanistic Nursing Theory, I received a phone call from a registered nurse from the mid-west. She was a graduate student taking her first course in nursing theory and had chosen the theory of Humanistic Nursing as the topic of her term paper. She was being discouraged by her instructor and dissuaded by some other academic nursing professionals that she had contacted. The reasons given ranged from lack of clarity of the theory, to not enough mention in the literature about clinical or research applications, to the assertion that Humanistic Nursing Theory is a theory that has "had its day." I have heard these criticisms before, both personally and related by other students. The purpose of the following chapter is to clarify these and other relevant issues. The applications presented in the second chapter are directed toward enhancing the understanding of the practical applications of Humanistic Nursing Theory.

As for Humanistic Nursing Theory having had its day, I still believe that it was before its time and it is only recently, in an atmosphere of theory-based nursing, that it is being received and understood in its full range of meaning. 'Why now?', you may ask, as this student did. I truly believe that it is related to the changing world view. There is an increasing acceptance of a world view that does not embrace the reductionist mind set as the touchstone of explanatory power. More and more there is an awareness of interrelatedness or, in terms of Humanistic Nursing Theory, the "all at once" quality of existence. It includes a temporal component which provides a space/time immediacy to the phenomenon in the "here and now." According to this view, patients and nurses bring all that they are, "all at once," as they engage in a dialogue that is the "essence" of nursing. It is a theory that does not reduce either the patient or the nurse to needs, pathology, or culture. It is an inclusive theory that provides a method for managing the complexities that are the reality of "being-in-the-world." At the same time it offers a means of prioritizing and focusing which allows for growth and enrichment. I will show how Humanistic Nursing Theory provides an umbrella, in other words, that it is a meta-theory, under which other nursing theories are subsumed and can be explained.

Questions that students of Humanistic Nursing Theory ask are not only related to the concepts and the application of the theory itself. There are also important questions about how we might use this newly found awareness and understanding of the "essential characteristics of nursing" to enhance nursing as a profession.

Martin Buber (1965) has eloquently said that humans have a basic need to be confirmed by others of their kind, "secretly and bashfully (they) watch for a "Yes" which allows (them) to be (p.71)." In Humanistic Nursing Theory we experience that "yes" as we encounter outward expression of that which we have inwardly known. We are uplifted by the "poiesis," the bringing-forth and bursting open of the blossom of possibilities that this brings (Heidegger, 1977, p. 10).

THE THEORISTS

Who are the theorists who authored Humanistic Nursing Theory? Dr. Josephine Paterson is originally from the east coast and Dr. Loretta Zderad is from the midwest. Each attended different diploma schools of nursing and different undergraduate programs, both receiving their bachelor's degree in Nursing Education. In their graduate work Dr. Zderad majored in psychiatric nursing at The Catholic University of America and Dr. Paterson in public health nursing at Johns Hopkins University. They met in the mid-fifties when they both worked at Catholic University. Their task was to create a new program that would encompass the community health component and the psychiatric component of the graduate program. That started a process of collaboration and dialogue and friendship that has lasted for over thirty-five years.

Dr. Zderad earned the PhD from Georgetown University and Dr. Paterson earned the DNSc from Boston University. Dr. Zderad's dissertation was on empathy and Dr. Paterson's was on comfort. They shared and developed their concepts, approaches, and experiences of "existential phenomenology" which evolved into the formal theory of Humanistic Nursing. They incorporated these into their work as educators and shared them across the country in seminars and workshops on Humanistic Nursing Theory. This theory may be considered a prototype for some of the more recent experiential based nursing theories (Benner, 1984; Parse, 1981; Watson, 1988).

My first contact with Humanistic Nursing Theory was when I was a graduate student in psychiatric mental health nursing. Josephine Paterson's name was given to me as a possible preceptor for my clinical placement. At that time Dr. Paterson was working as a Psychotherapist at the Veterans Hospital in Northport, Long Island in the Mental Hygiene Clinic and was also Adjunct Associate Professor at Adelphi University. Loretta Zderad was at that time, the Associate Chief of Nursing Service for Education at the same Veterans Hospital.

Dr. Paterson and Dr. Zderad came to the Veterans Administration Hospital in Northport in 1971. They were hired for their original positions as nursologists by a forward thinking administrator who recognized the need for staff support during a period of change in the VA system. The position of nursologist involved a three pronged approach to the improvement of patient care through clinical practice, education, and research. These functions were integrated within the framework of Humanistic Nursing. They worked with the nurses at Northport in this manner from 1971 until 1978. At that time they assumed the positions which they held when I met them.

My initial interview with Dr. Paterson went well and she agreed to work with me over the next two years. Perhaps she had an attraction to the "all at onceness" of my multidimensional life. At that time, I was working full time, a graduate student, a wife, a mother, and a homemaker. I am eternally grateful to her for those sunrise hours of supervision before I went off to work. The following week I had the privilege of meeting Loretta Zderad.

When I first met Dr. Paterson and Dr. Zderad, I had no awareness of Humanistic Nursing Theory. During our discussions however, it became apparent that we shared an interest in certain writers. For example, we spoke about Martin Buber and the "I and Thou" concept and "dialogue" as the process of intersubjective relating. We also spoke about Rollo May (1975) and his work on creativity. At some point Dr. Paterson casually mentioned that I might be interested in reading a book that she and Dr. Zderad had written. She indicated that the book referenced these writers as well as some Existentialists such as Marcel, Desan, and Popper. The book was *Humanistic Nursing* (1988). The following two years brought me a world of enrichment. For Dr. Paterson and Dr. Zderad the next two years culminated in their retirement and relocation to the south. I, on the other hand, continue the work that they started, as a fellow theorist, and as a friend and colleague in nursing.

Since their retirement, Dr. Zderad and Dr. Paterson refer inquiries about Humanistic Nursing Theory to me. The reasons for this honor I have been told are that they believe I have "a real grasp of what the theory is about." They also appreciate how alive it is in my everyday practice of nursing. It has given me the opportunity to speak individually to students or to present and discuss the theory with groups of nurses. At these times I am aware of the disappointment that nurses feel in not being able to have more direct access to the theorists themselves. I feel privileged to have had a professional and a personal relationship in which I have been able to dialogue with Dr. Paterson and Dr. Zderad about Humanistic Nursing Theory. With this privilege I also experience a responsibility to share what that dialogue has offered me. I do, however, have concerns when they refer people to me that I represent Humanistic Nursing Theory accurately and adequately.

My call to Dr. Paterson and Dr. Zderad for validation of my representation of their theory in discourse and in writing has been responded to with confirmation that I have done what they had hoped nurses would do (Kleiman, 1985). That is I have taken Humanistic Nursing Theory and made it my own, expanded it, and articulated it to others. And so while I may use a different style, and in our world scholars at times may differ, I am confident based on their validation that the core concepts of the theory have not been distorted. Perhaps my particular contribution is that I have taken the basic theoretical concepts of Humanistic Nursing Theory which were originally articulated and conceptualized through the shared experiences of nurses, and shown how nurses can use those concepts to expand and enrich themselves, their patients, nursing, and health care in general. Dr. Paterson and Dr. Zderad's response to my call was that it was now our theory. "Our theory" to me meaning a theory in progress, to be owned, expanded upon, and hopefully articulated by all those nurses who embrace it as their own.

REFERENCES

Benner, P. (1984). *From novice to expert*. Menlo Park, CA: Addison-Wesley Publishing Co.

Buber, M. (1965). *The knowledge of man*. New York: Harper & Row Publishers, Inc.

Heidegger, M. (1977). *The question concerning technology*. New York: Harper & Row Publishers, Inc.

May, R. (1975). *The courage to create*. New York: Norton.

Parse, R. (19B1). *Man-living-health: A theory of nursing*. New York: John Wiley & Sons.

Paterson, J. G., & Zderad, L. T. (1988). *Humanistic Nursing*. New York: National League for Nursing Press.

Watson, J. (1988). *Nursing: Human science and human care*. New York: National League for Nursing Press.

3

Humanistic Nursing Theory

Susan Kleiman

Humanistic Nursing Theory is multidimensional. It speaks to the essences of nursing and embraces the dynamics of being, becoming, and change. It is an interactive theory of nursing which provides a methodology for reflective articulation of nursing essences. It is also a theory that provides a methodological bridge between theory and practice by providing a broad guide for nursing "dialogue" in a myriad of settings.

Nursing as seen through Humanistic Nursing Theory is the ability to struggle with another through "peak experiences related to health and suffering in which the participants in the nursing situation are and become in accordance with their human potential" (Paterson & Zderad, 1976, p. 7). The struggle is shared through a dialogue between the participants. This mandate to share "struggles with," is what allows for each to "become" in relationship with the other. In nursing, the purpose of this dialogue, or intersubjective relating, according to Josephine Paterson and Loretta Zderad is, "Nurturing the well-being and more-being of persons in need" (p. 4). Humanistic Nursing Theory is grounded in existentialism and emphasizes the lived experience of nursing. One of the existential themes that it builds on is the affirmation of being and becoming of both the patient and the nurse through the choices they make and the intersubjective relationships they engage in. This dynamic is expressed as nursing's concern with the struggle toward self-actualizing potential or "more-being."

The new adventurer in humanistic nursing theory may at first find some of these terms and phrases awkward. When I spoke to a colleague of the "moreness" and of "relating all-at-once" she remarked, "Oh, oh, you're beginning to sound just like them," meaning Dr. Paterson and Dr. Zderad. What was of note to her, has become natural to me. It is reflective of my grasp of nursing as an ever changing process. Think of your nursing experiences, whatever the contexts may be. Are these experiences of static settings? Or is there a pervasive sense of activity associated with them? Just as nursing in actual practice is never inert, so Humanistic Nursing Theory is in its essence dynamic. I reflect with a smile on Josephine Paterson's description of humanistic nursing, "Our 'here and now' stage of humanistic nursing practice theory development at times is experienced as an all-at-once octopus at a discotheque, stimulation personified gyrating in many colors" (1977, p. 4). It is a bonus when a theory can not only be useful but can also be fun.

While this approach to theory may seem somewhat lighthearted, it addresses the need to feel comfortable with theory. Theory like research, is not just for those in ivory towers. Theory and research are a part of every nurse and all that is nursing. If we look at theory through R. D. Lang's eyes as "an articulated vision of experience" (Zderad, 1978a, p. 4) we can see that in one sense by looking at our own experience of nursing, as proposed in Humanistic Nursing Theory, we all become theorists. I do not use the term, "comfortable with" in the generic sense, but rather in the humanistic nursing sense. Comfort in this view is that which allows persons to be all that they can be in particular lived situations. Theory should offer nurses comfort in their everyday nursing. In other words, theory should offer nurses assistance to be all that they can be in their particular lived nursing situations.

If I were asked to succinctly conceptualize humanistic nursing theory I would have to say, "call and response." These three words encapsulate for me the core themes of this quite elegant and very profound theory. In what follows, you will come to understand that through this paradigm, Josephine Paterson and Loretta Zderad have presented a vision of nursing that withstands variation in practice settings and the changing patterns of nursing over time.

According to Humanistic Nursing Theory, there is a call from a person, a family, a community, or from humanity for help with some health related issue. A nurse, a group of nurses, or the community of nurses hearing and recognizing that call responds in a manner that is

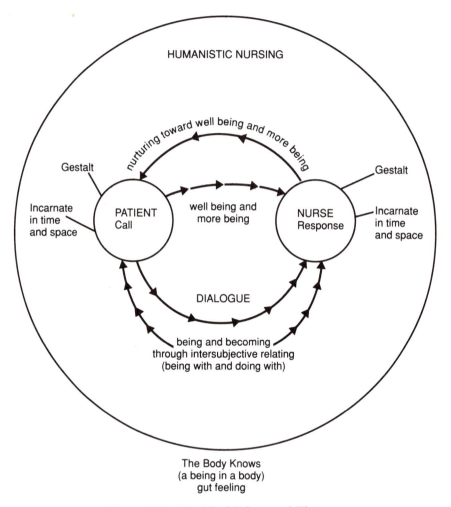

Figure 3.1   World of Others and Things.

intended to help the caller with the health related need. What happens during this dialogue, the "and" in the "call-and-response," the "between," is nursing.

In their book, *Humanistic Nursing* (1976), Drs. Paterson and Zderad share with other nurses their method for exploring the "between," again emphasizing that it is the "between" that they conceive of as nursing. The method is phenomenological inquiry (Paterson & Zderad, p. 72).

Engaging in phenomenological inquiry sensitizes the inquiring nurse to the excitement, fear, and uncertainty of approaching the nursing situation openly. Through a spirit of receptivity, a readiness for surprise, and the courage to experience the unknown there is an opportunity for authentic relatedness and intersubjectvity. "The process leads one naturally to repeated experiencing of and reflective immersion in the lived phenomena" (Zderad, 1978, p. 8). This immersion into the intersubjective experience and the phenomenological process that one engages in helps guide the nurse in the responsive interchange between the patient and the nurse. During this interchange the nurse calls forth all that she is (education, skills, life experiences, etc.) and integrates it into her response. A common misconception that some students of Humanistic Nursing Theory have is that it asserts that the nurse must provide what it is that the patient is calling for. Remember the response of the nurse is guided by all that she is. This includes her professional role, ethics, and competencies. And so while a response may not actually provide what is being called for, the process of being heard according to this theory is in itself a humanizing experience.

This explanation of humanistic nursing theory calls for elaboration of some of its basic concepts and assumptions. Let's look at the conceptual framework of Humanistic Nursing Theory represented in the preceding diagram (see Figure 3.1).

Humanistic nursing is a moving process that occurs in the living context of human beings, human beings who interface and interact with others and other things in the world. This conceptual framework represents a nonlinear process that, over time, spirals upward. This fluidity may be somewhat disturbing to the beginning explorer of Humanistic Nursing Theory. It is this fluidity however that once grasped, allows for the generalization to a diversity of practice settings.

In the world of Humanistic Nursing Theory the human beings identified are the patient (i.e., person, family, community, or humanity) and the nurse (Figure 3.2). A patient becomes identified as the patient when he sends a call for help with some health related problem. The person hearing and recognizing the call is the nurse. The nurse is another human being who by intentionally choosing to become a nurse has made a commitment to help others in relation to their health needs.

It is important to emphasize that the nurse and the patient are both first human beings, or groups of human beings with their own particular

Nursing is Transactional

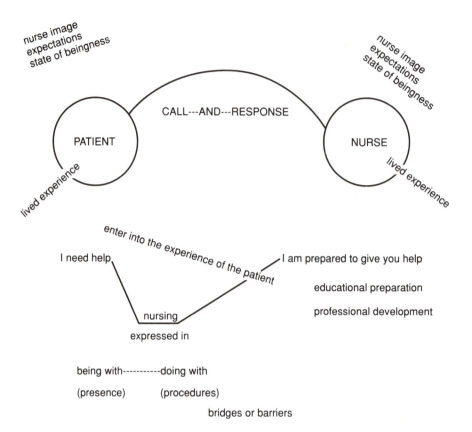

Figure 3.2 Shared Human Experience.

gestalts (Figure 3.3). Gestalt, representing all that those human beings are, includes all their past experiences, all their current being, and all their hopes, dreams, and fears of the future which are experienced in their own space/time dimension. This includes the environmental resources available to them, factors that have increasing import in times of fiscal constraints. In sum, using a humanistic nursing term, they exist "all-at-once." In the context of nursing, when these two human beings encounter and interact with each other, that interaction centers on the call from one person, the patient, for a helpful response from another, the nurse. While the call and response is between the nurse and the

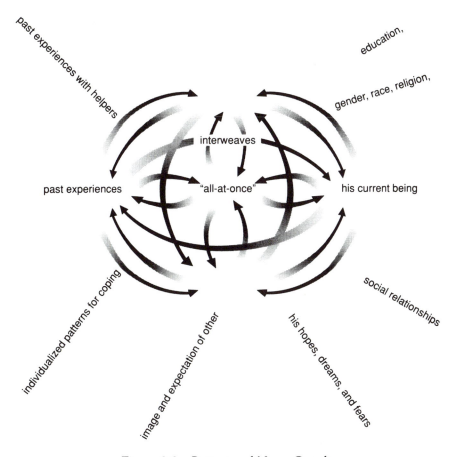

Figure 3.3 Patient and Nurse Gestalts.

patient, it is important to understand that all else that makes this particular person who they are enters in this interaction too.

This gestalt includes the patient's past and current social relationships, such as the experiences of gender, race, religion, as well as education, work, and whatever individualized patterns for coping with the experience of living have developed. It also includes past experiences with helpers in the health care system and the patient's image and expectation of what it is that they are calling to the nurse for. As incarnate human beings we exist in this particular space at this particular time in a physical body that senses, filters, and processes our experiences.

The nurse too brings all that she is. Her expectation is however, that she be able to respond to the call for help as a nurse. The nurse then interweaves her professional identity and professional education, with all her other life experiences to create her own tapestry which she projects through her nursing responses. One has only to observe nurses going about their nursing to see how individualized the expressed dialogue with a particular patient can be. A very simple example of this may be two nurses performing the same task of suctioning a patient. Depending on the nurse and the patient I have seen this done with tenderness, with humor, and with masterful technical skills that make the procedure almost unnoticeable. I noticed one nurse that each time she positioned and suctioned the person she was working with, made sure that she also repositioned the little basket of flowers that the nurse had placed by the patient's bedside. It is this individuality as human beings that makes us alike and which provides one of the threads that unite us throughout this process of living. Being alike in our differences is only one of those core threads however, and in nursing, humanistic theory attempts to uncover the other unifying threads or essences that make up the human fabric of nursing. The nurse must always be aware that since in existential theory human beings become through the choices they make and the intersubjective experiences they engage in, the choice to intersubjectively engage and the level of that intersubjective relating is mutually determined by the patient and nurse.

PHILOSOPHICAL AND
METHODOLOGICAL BACKGROUND

The phenomenological movement of the nineteenth century was in response to what its proponents called the dehumanization and objectification of the world by the scientific community. Phenomenologists proposed that human beings, the world, and their experiences of their world are inseparable. You can easily see that a nursing theory that is based in the human context lends itself to phenomenological inquiry rather than reductionism which attempts to remove subjective humanness and strives to achieve detached objectivity. The early phenomenologists saw their goal as the examination and description of all things including the human experience of those things, in the particular way that they reveal themselves without preconceived ideas or assumptions. In the early 1960's Josephine Paterson and Loretta Zderad gravitated toward this method to first examine their own nursing. Later they used this method to work with other nurses in examining their nursing practice to explicate its essences. Today, nursing phenomenologists use variations of phenomenological methods to examine the experiential phenomena of nursing.

There are people however, who profess that phenomenology is not a philosophy but is at best a method—a method developed by applying phenonomenological concepts. In other words phenomenology is the "experience" of a method which can be integrated into a general approach or way of viewing the world. As I mentioned before, nurses who can relate to this method are inclined to cultivate it and make it a part of their everyday approach to nursing. This method is no less rigorous in its application than the method used in experimental research to build theories. The phenomenological approach is based on description, intuition, analysis, and synthesis. Intuitive openness and accurate description require some aptitude for this conceptual framework. Of importance are training and conscientious self-criticism on the part of the unbiased inquirer as the inquirer investigates the phenomenon as it reveals itself. In phenomenology a statement's validity is based on whether or not it describes the phenomena accurately. The truth of all the premises resulting from the critical analysis of the described phenomenon can be verified by examining the phenomena itself.

Dr. Paterson and Dr. Zderad describe five phases to their phenomenological study of nursing. These phases are presented sequentially but actually in this process they are interwoven, since as with all of Humanistic Nursing Theory there is a constant flow between, in all directions, and all-at-once emanating toward a center that is nursing. The phases of humanistic nursing inquiry are:

- Preparation of the nurse knower for coming to know
- Nurse knowing the other intuitively
- Nurse knowing the other scientifically
- Nurse complementarily synthesizing known others
- Succession within the nurse from the many to the paradoxical one

Enfolded in these five phases are three concepts that are very basic to Humanistic Nursing Theory. They are: bracketing, angular view, and noetic loci. These will be taken up as we discuss the phases of inquiry.

Preparation of the Nurse Knower for Coming to Know

In the first phase the inquirer tries to open herself up to the unknown and possibly different. She consciously and conscientiously struggles with understanding and identifying her own "angular view." Angular view involves the gestalt of the human that we spoke about earlier. It includes the conceptual and experiential framework that we bring into any situation with us which are usually unexamined and casually accepted as we negotiate our every day world. Angular view is not judged. It is a component of the process and needs to be recognized as such. Later in the process it is called upon to help make sense of and give meaning to the experience of inquiry.

By identifying our angular view we are then able to purposefully bracket it so that we do not superimpose it on the experience we are trying to relate to. When we bracket, we purposefully hold our own thoughts, experiences, and beliefs in abeyance. I re-emphasize that this abeyance does not deny our unique selves but suspends them, allowing us to experience the other in their own uniqueness. This is primary to phenomenological inquiry which calls on us to see that which the phenomena reveals itself in itself to be. If you will think for a moment about a line from an old Paul Simon song, "A man hears what he wants to hear and disregards the rest." This is what bracketing tries to avoid. Using this metaphor, the phenomenological approach requires us to hear, "what a man wants to say and to temporarily disregard the rest."*

By becoming aware of and acknowledging what we think is true we can then attempt to hold these assumptions in abeyance so that they will not prematurely intrude upon one's attempts to describe the experiences of another. A personal experience that helped me to grasp the concept of bracketing occurred a few years ago when I was traveling in Europe. As I entered each new country, I experienced the excitement of the unknown. I realized, at the same time how alert, open and other directed I was in this uncharted world as compared to my own daily routine at home. Here at times I would kind of fill in the blanks left by

---

*Lyrics from *The Boxer* by Paul Simon, copyright © 1968 Paul Simon. Used by permission of the publisher.

my inattentiveness to a routine experience, sometimes anticipating and answering questions even before they were asked. This alertness, openness, and other directedness is the goal of bracketing. According to Husserl (1970), who is considered the father of modern phenomenology, the state desired is that of the perpetual beginner.

Bracketing prepares the inquirer to enter the uncharted world of the other without expectations and preconceived ideas. It helps one to be open to the authentic, in other words the true, experience of the other. Even temporarily letting go of that which shapes our own identity as the self however, causes anxiety, fear, and uncertainty. Labeling, diagnosing, and routines add a necessary and very valuable predictability, sense of security, and a means of conserving energy to our everyday existence and practice. It however may also make us less open to the new and different in a situation. Being open to the new and different is a necessary stance in being able to know of the other intuitively.

Nurse Knowing the Other Intuitively

Knowing the other intuitively is described by Dr. Paterson and Dr. Zderad as "moving back and forth between the impressions the nurse becomes aware of in herself and the recollected real experience of the other" (1976, p. 88–89) which was obtained through the unbiased being with the other. This is not a contradictory process of bracketing versus intuiting. They are both necessary and interwoven parts of the phenomenological process. The rigor and validity of phenomenology is based on the on-going referring back to the phenomenon itself. It is conceptualized as a dialectic between the impression and the real. This shifting back and forth allows for sudden insights on the part of the nurse, a new overall grasp which manifests itself in a clearer or perhaps a new "understanding of." These understandings generate further development of the process. At this time the nurse's general impressions are in a dialogue with her unbracketed view (Figure 3.4).

Nurse Knowing the Other Scientifically

In the next phase, objectivity is needed as the nurse comes to know the other scientifically. Standing outside the phenomenon the nurse examines it through analysis. She comes to know it through its parts or elements that are symbolic and known. This phase incorporates the nurse's ability to be conscious of herself and that which she has taken

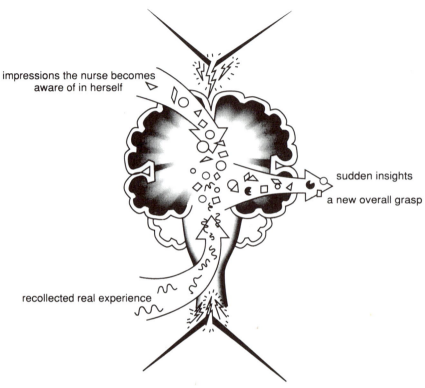

impressions the nurse becomes
aware of in herself

sudden insights

a new overall grasp

recollected real experience

At this time the nurse's general impressions
are in a dialogue with her unbracketed view

Adapted from illustration in Briggs, J. & Peat, D. (1989). *Turbulent Mirror*, New York: Harper & Row Publishers, p. 176.

Figure 3.4   Nurse knowing the other intuitively.

in, merged with, made part of herself. "This is the time when the nurse mulls over, analyzes, sorts out, compares, contrasts, relates, interprets, gives a name to, and categorizes" (Paterson & Zderad, p. 79). Patterns and themes are reflective of and rigorously validated by the authentic experience (Figure 3.5).

Nurse Complementarily Synthesizing Known Others

At this point the nurse personifies what has been described by Dr. Paterson and Dr. Zderad as a "noetic locus" a "knowing place" (1976,

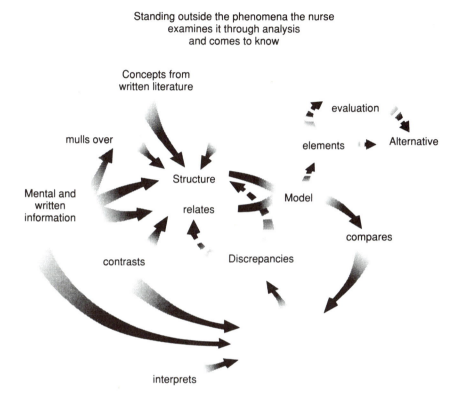

Standing outside the phenomena the nurse
examines it through analysis
and comes to know

Concepts from
written literature

mulls over

evaluation

elements   Alternative

Mental and
written
information

Structure

relates   Model

compares

contrasts   Discrepancies

interprets

nurse conscious of herself

Adapted from illustration in Briggs, J. & Peat, D. (1989). *Turbulent Mirror*, New York: Harper & Row Publishers, p. 176.

Figure 3.5   Nurse knowing the other scientifically.

p. 43). According to this concept the greatest gift a human being can have is the ability to relate to others, to wonder, search and imagine about experience, and to create out of what has become known. The ability of nurses to see themselves as "knowing places" encourages them to continue to develop their community of world thinkers through their educative processes which then becomes a part of their angular view. This self expansion through the internalization of what others have come to know, dynamically interrelates with the nurse's human capacity to be conscious of their own lived experiences. Through this interrelationship the subjective and objective world of nursing can be re-

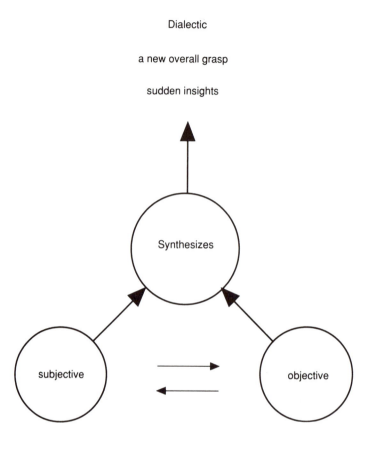

Figure 3.6 Nurse complementarily synthesizing known others.

flected upon by each nurse, who is aware of and values herself as a "knowing place" (Figure 3.6).

Succession within the Nurse
from the Many to the Paradoxical One

This is the birth of the new from the existing patterns, themes, and categories. It is in this phase that the nurse "comes up with a conception or abstraction that is inclusive of and beyond the multiplicities and contradictions" (Paterson & Zderad, 1976, p. 81), in a process that corrects and expands her own angular view.

This is the pattern of the dialectic process which is reflected throughout humanistic nursing theory. In the dialectic process there is a repetitive pattern of organizing the dissimilar into a higher level (Barnum, 1989, p. 44). At this higher level differences are assimilated to create the new. This repetitive dialectic process of humanistic nursing is an approach that feels comfortable and natural for those who think inductively. For me the pervasive theme of dialectic assimilation speaks to universal interrelatedness from the simplest to the most complex level. Human beings by virtue of their ability to be self-observing have the unique capacity to transcend themselves and dialectically reflect on their relationship to the universe. This dialectic process has a pattern similar to that of the call and response paradigm of Humanistic Nursing Theory. This paradigm speaks to the interactive dialogue between two different human beings from which a unique, yet universal instance of nursing emerges. The nursing interaction is limited in time and space but the internalization of that experience adds something new to each person's angular view. Neither are the same as before. Each is more because of that coming together. The coming together of the nurse and the patient, the between in the lived world, is nursing. Just as in the double helix of the DNA molecule, this interweaving pattern is what structures the individual. In the fabric of humanistic nursing theory this intentional interweaving between patient and nurse is what also gives nursing its structure, form, and meaning.

Dr. Paterson and Dr. Zderad used this method of phenomenological inquiry and dialectic synthesis in workshops with other nurses. Over 2000 descriptions of nursing were written by more than 120 nurses who shared their lived world of nursing with each other. From the analysis and synthesis of these descriptions eleven phenomena of nursing were generated. These are: awareness, openness, empathy, caring, touching, understanding, responsibility, trust, acceptance, self-recognition, and dialogue. These phenomena were envisioned as the constants in the ever-changing world of patient and nurse interaction.

THE CONCEPT OF COMMUNITY

The definition of community presented by Drs. Paterson and Zderad is, "Two or more persons struggling together toward a center" (1976,

p. 131). They and the other nurses from their workshops were very much a community, a community of nurses struggling toward a center that is nursing. Just as in any community there is the individual and the collective known as the community. Plato points to the microcosm and the macrocosm and proposes that the one is reflective of the many. In unification theories the emphasis is on recurrent patterns that given enough distance would be found in all the universe. Humanistic Nursing Theory can be considered both a micro and macro theory in which the nursing interaction of one is considered to be a reflection of the recurrent pattern of nursing and is therefore worth reflecting upon and valuing. All nurses are members of a community of nurses struggling toward a center that is nursing through dialogue and interaction. A distinguishing concept of Humanistic Nursing Theory is an inherent obligation of nurses to each other in this community. That which enhances one of us, enhances all of us. Through openness, sharing, and caring we each will expand our angular views, each becoming more than before. Subsequently we take back into our nursing community these expanded selves which in turn will touch our patients, other colleagues, and the world of health care.

REFERENCES

Barnum, B. J. S. (1990). *Nursing theory: Analysis, application, evaluation.* Glenview, IL: Scott, Foresman, Co.

Husserl, L. (1970). *The idea of phenomenology.* The Hague: Martinus Nijhoff.

Paterson, J. G. (1977). Living until death, my perspective. Paper presented at the Syracuse Veteran's Administration Hospital, New York.

Paterson, J. G., & Zderad, L. T. (1976). *Humanistic nursing.* New York: John Wiley & Sons.

Simon, P. (1969). *The Boxer.* New York: Columbia Records.

4

Clinical Applications of Humanistic Nursing Theory

Susan Kleiman

NURSE'S REFLECTION ON NURSING

As an introduction to the clinical applications of Humanistic Nursing Theory, I will share with you two explorations from Dr. Paterson's and Dr. Zderad's nursing experiences. These descriptive explorations are related to the concepts of empathy, comfort, and presence. Dr. Paterson (1977) shared her experiences with a terminally ill cancer patient. She describes, "For a while I really beat on myself. I felt nothing, just a kind of indifference and numbness, as Dominic expressed his miseries, fears, and anger. I pride myself on my empathic ability. I felt so inadequate. I could not believe I could not feel with him what he was experiencing. Intellectually I knew his words, his expressions were pain-filled. My feelings of inadequacy, helplessness, and inability to control myself, came through strong. I mulled reflectively about this, suddenly a light dawned amidst my puzzlement. I was experiencing what Dominic was expressing. At this time I was feeling his inadequacy, helplessness, and inability to control his cancer" (p. 13).

This insight brought a greater understanding between Dr. Paterson and this patient, an understanding that brought them closer so that she could endure with him in his fear-filled knowing and unknowing of dying. As his condition deteriorated she continued to visit at his bedside. "Often after greeting me and saying what he needed he would fall asleep. First, I thought, 'It doesn't matter whether I come or not.' Then

I noticed and validated that when I moved his eyes flew open. I reevaluated his sleeping during my visit. I discussed this with him. He felt safe when I sat with him. He was exhausted, staying awake, watching himself to be sure he did not die. When I was there I watched him, and he could sleep. I no longer made any move to leave before my time with him was up. I told him of this intention, so that he could relax more deeply. To alleviate aloneness; this is a most expensive gift. To give this gift of time, and presence in the patient's space, a person has to value, the outcomes of relating."

This gift of presence is poetically described by Dr. Zderad (1978, p. 48):

> Death lifts his scythe
>   to swipe down the young man
>   misdressed in hospital gown
>   displaced in hospital bed.
>
> The cruel cold blade slashes
>   the hard mask of his nurse
>   silently standing there
>   bleeding forth her presence.

The beauty of the articulation of this essence is that it encourages other nurses to reflect, value, and further communicate the essences of their practice. And so Dr. Paterson's and Dr. Zderad's accounts brought back to mind an experience of mine that had stayed with me for years but that I had not truly reflected upon until exposed to the process of humanistic nursing.

Years ago I worked on the night shift in the nursing home portion of a hospital center. One of the patients I worked with was Mrs. W., an eighty-four year old woman who had a major stroke two years before as well as several serious infections during that time. Mrs. W. was becoming increasingly compromised in her ability to move and provide any of her own self-care.

Some of the staff had difficulty with Mrs. W. and described her as ornery, nasty, and demanding. She was known to scratch and pull hair if she was displeased with the way she was being positioned during the night. She could speak, but would do so sparingly and seemed to be able to express herself best with four letter words.

One night as I walked through the rooms checking on the patients at the beginning of the shift, I experienced something different immediately upon entering Mrs. W.'s room. It was intuitive. I wasn't sure what it was at first, but upon making eye contact with her I again immediately felt a different sense of connectedness between us. I walked closer and was able to sense a welcoming engagement and a previously not present softness about her. I instinctively touched her hand and she did not respond in her usual combative manner, as somehow I knew she wouldn't. I asked her how she was feeling, and with a barely visible smile, she said softly, "Oh, okay, but do you think I could stay for awhile?" I said, "Of course, you can stay as long as you like." I then told her I'd be back. I went to her chart and there was nothing different noted, but there was something different. I went back and casually did her vital signs, which were all within normal limits for her. There seemed to be no physical indication that she was in any distress. I knew something was happening though. I felt that she was getting ready to leave.

I made it a point to spend a lot of time with Mrs. W. that night, fortunately it was not particularly busy. She let me comb her hair and fuss with her a bit. While I did this she pointed to the picture of her family and for the first time shared some family stories with me. As I was leaving to go home I stopped in to say goodbye to Mrs. W. She put her hand on mine and weakly smiled goodbye. And I knew we were really saying goodbye for good. Something special had happened between us so instead of feeling badly we both seemed to feel quietly good.

Mrs. W. died two hours later. It may seem bizarre, but I smiled when I heard. I was glad that we had spent so much time together the night before. I truly believe that I helped Mrs. W. with her inevitable passage with my presence. I know she helped me to experience dying as something that at times is quietly welcome by allowing me to be with her at the beginning of that passage.

Upon reflecting and trying to understand this experience of the patient I have become better able to share in the final journeys of others. By being with her in her experience she has given me a better understanding of how to offer comfort to those that are dying. I thank her for our experience.

PATIENT'S REFLECTION ON NURSING

It is of great interest to me when I come across reflections by patients of their experiences with nurses. These reflective experiences also help to clarify the essences of nursing. Two years ago I attended a conference on "Love, intimacy, and connectedness." It was an interdisciplinary conference attended by three to four hundred people.

One of the opening speakers described the experience that had been related to him by a dear friend. This experience related to his friend just being diagnosed with a serious form of cancer. He describes his friend telling him, "In the early evening the family was all around. We talked but there was the awkwardness of not knowing what to say or what to expect. Later that night, I was in my room all alone. No longer having to be concerned about my family and what they were struggling with, I began to experience some of my own feelings. I felt so alone. Then the evening nurse who had been working with me over the last two days of testing came in. We looked at each other, neither of us said a word and she just gently touched my hand. I cried. She stayed there for, I don't know how long, until I placed my other hand on top of hers and gently gave it a pat. She left and I was able to go to sleep. This was one of the most intimate moments in my life. This nurse offered to be with me in the known and somehow she also conveyed a reassurance that I did not have to go through what was coming, whatever that was, alone."

This ability to be with and endure with the patient in their process of living is frequently taken for granted by us and yet it is what many times differentiates us from other professionals. In my practice as nursing care coordinator I frequently engage in the phenomenological process of humanistic nursing to help me in my everyday interactions. On one occasion the department heads of the day hospital where I work were talking about a program evaluation. This evaluation was partially a result of a study that the nurses of the day hospital had done. I was proposing that it was important to have patients share with us their experience of the groups that they attended. One of the doctors of the day hospital voiced his skepticism that the patients' input was actually necessary. He said that after all he was aware of their pathology and diagnosis. Based on this he believed he could judge the effectiveness of a group by using his clinical skills to assess changes in symptomatology. I took exception to this and must admit I got a little hot under the collar. Upon reflecting on this experience, however, I had an insight related to the angular view. I realized that this doctor was coming from the angular view of medicine rather than the angular view of nursing which emphasizes that the patients' views and experiences are primary to the treatment process. I felt more tolerant of this doctor at that point. But more important, I had an experience of the difference between doctoring and nursing. Nurses must recognize the difference, respect these differences in the health care field, and accept the responsibility of meeting the challenges to nursing that those differences entail.

USES OF THE THEORY IN CLINICAL SUPERVISION

In my clinical supervision with the nurses in the day hospital I use the humanistic nursing approach. In the process of supervision I try to understand the "call" of the nurse when she brings up a clinical issue. This usually is connected to the "call" of the patient to her and some issue that has arisen around the nurse's not being able to hear or respond to that call.

An illustration of this can be seen in one of my nurse supervising experiences. Ms. L. was working with a patient who had recently been told that her HIV test was positive. While she did not have AIDS she was exposed to the AIDS virus, probably through her current boyfriend, who was purportedly an I.V. drug abuser. The original issue that came up was that the nurse was very concerned that the doctor on the interdisciplinary team, who was also the patient's therapist, was not giving the patient the support that the nurse felt the patient was calling out for. This nurse and I explored her perception that the patient did in fact seem to be reaching out. The nurse and I explored the reaching out in terms of what the patient was reaching for. It had been carefully explained to the patient that she did not have AIDS, but at some point she might come down with the illness. At that time she was told that there were treatments to retard the disease but as of now there were no cures. Given this, the doctor whose primary function is treatment and cure, was feeling ill prepared to deal with this patient and it was perhaps this sense of inadequacy that fostered avoidant behavior on his part. The nurse and I, however, came to understand that in fact, the patient was not calling for doctoring, she was calling for nursing care. She was calling for someone to help her get through this experience in her life. When this was clarified, the nurse and I began to explore the nurse's experience of hearing this call. The nurse spoke of the pain of knowing that this young woman who was close to her own age would die prematurely. She spoke of how a friend, who reminded her of this patient, had also died and that when she associated the two she felt sad. This nurse also had had some difficult personal experiences which she touched upon which elicited a will to survive, which she also could relate to this patient.

As we explored what really was the nurse's angular view we were able to identify areas that were unknown. She had difficulty understanding the need or the role of the relationship with her current boyfriend. We worked on helping the nurse to bracket her own thoughts and judgments so that she could be open to the patient's experience of this relationship. Subsequently the nurse was able to understand the patient's intense fear of being alone. The nurse's understanding that choices are humanizing, now began to explore the need for support systems. In the experience of her own angular view, as a part of her being her own "knowing place," the nurse realized that she herself had things to learn in this area. And so to expand her own capability of being a "knowing place" and expanding her angular view, she sought out the help of the nurse practitioner in our gynecology clinic. They worked well together with this patient who eventually was able to leave our day hospital, get a part time job, and be all that she could in her current life situation.

The nurse in the day hospital grew from her experience of working with this patient. Although she is usually quite reserved and shies away from public forums, with encouragement she was able to share the experience with this patient in a large public forum. She not only shared with other professionals the role that she as a nurse played in the treatment of this patient, she also acknowledged herself in a group of professionals as a "knowing place." As for me, I was touched by this nurse's experience of struggling through this difficult situation to become more in her nursing realm and I became more because of her growth.

Another example of the application of Humanistic Nursing Theory in clinical practice involves a nurse working with a patient diagnosed with chronic schizophrenia. The patient had experienced several severe psychotic breaks with subsequent deterioration in functioning. In certain patients with schizophrenia who experience this downward course, it is heartbreaking to the patient and the family alike. In my supervision with this nurse, it became clear that she was struggling with the threatened decompensation of this patient each time discharge came near. She felt frustrated and at first like the patient was failing. Later she began to see that it was the team that was projecting their own sense of failure at not being able to get the patient to follow through with their discharge plan. By helping this nurse to relate and reflect upon her experience with this patient, she was able to see that he was not non-compliant, one of our favorite labels. When she was with the patient she began to see how hard he really was trying. When asked what she thought he might be calling to her for in their interactions she suddenly became aware that he was looking for someone to acknowledge how hard he was trying and that he didn't want to disappoint anyone but it was the best he could do.

The nurse with this new understanding, became aware of her need to validate to the patient that she understood. Her further nursing action was to take this information back to the team to help them recognize their own inability to deal with the patient's loss of functioning. For if they were unable to recognize it and deal with it how could they help the patient to deal with it? Subsequently both the nurse's actions and the team's actions were more in response to the patient's call rather than their own expectations and needs. This effected not only the attitude of the staff toward the patient but it also permitted them to make an appropriate discharge plan that the patient could follow through with. This nurse had the experience of herself as a "knowing place." She exerted her influence with new confidence in her interactions with the team. I, as her supervisor had a renewed experience in the validity of the process of humanistic nursing.

While the examples of clinical supervision I have cited were in the psychiatric setting, I do believe using the process enfolded in humanistic nursing theory is beneficial to supervisors and self-reflective practitioners in all areas of nursing. Patients call to us with all sorts of health related needs both verbally and nonverbally. It is important to hear the calls and know the process that lets us understand them. In hearing the calls and searching our own experiences of who we are, our personal angular view, we may progress as humanistic nurses.

USE OF THE THEORY IN RESEARCH

Shifting the application of the theory from the individual nurse to a community of nurses, I would like to share with you a group research project that was conducted in the clinical setting of a psychiatric day hospital. In an effort to better understand why some patients stayed in

the day hospital and others left, the nursing staff conducted a phenomenological study that investigated the experiences of patients as they
enter and become engaged in treatment in a day hospital system. The
initial step in the process, in Dr. Paterson's and Dr. Zderad's terms, is
to prepare the nurse knower for coming to know.

Part of the process of preparing the nurses for this study was to
expand their angular view by educating them in the phenomenological
method and the unstructured interview style. Literature was handed out
on this and meetings were held to discuss the articles and any questions
about them. We also shared our feelings about this method, our concerns, and other experiences related to this study. As we did this we
began to establish an atmosphere of openness and trust. This open atmosphere was essential to the preparation for gathering descriptions of
the patients' experiences. In order to further promote the openness of
the interviewers to the experience of the patients, we used our group
nursing meetings for the purpose of bracketing our angular views. In
these group meetings we raised our consciousness through articulation
of our own angular views. In addition, by opening ourselves to each
other's experiences and points of view we were opening ourselves to the
world of other possibilities and shaking up the status quo of our own
mind sets. Once the descriptions were obtained, we as a group interpreted with the phenomenological method of reflecting, intuiting, analyzing, and synthesizing. We interviewed fifteen patients over a period
of eight months, on their day of admission and every four weeks there-
after until discharge.

A brief example of the outcome of this study was that from our
interviews we found that there were many anxiety producing experiences on the first day in the day hospital, but very few anxiety reducing
experiences that offered the patient comfort and support. The two patients that left the study at this time found no anxiety reducing experiences at all. Subsequently recommendations were made that were
hypothesized to reduce the anxiety of the patient on the first day. This
is an example of how through this method hypotheses are generated
that can then be tested in the scientific method.

The concept of research as praxis is also illustrated in this research
project. On an individual basis the nurses related that they experienced
an increased awareness of the need to be open to the patients' expressions of themselves. The nurses also expressed that they now felt that
they had an awareness of a comfortable method that would help them

with this openness as well as a method for analyzing the experience to gain a better understanding of the phenomenon.

After reviewing the interviews of a patient who had had a particularly difficult course of treatment, one of the nurses who was on her treatment team remarked, "We weren't listening to what she was telling us—we just didn't hear the pain." Another nurse had a similar insight into a patient's experiences. She noted with some surprise that her initial impression that a patient she was working with was hostile and withholding had given way to the realization that this patient as a result of the negative symptoms of schizophrenia was quite empty and was really giving us all that she had to give. The nurse in future interactions with this patient was empathic and supportive rather than judgmental and angry.

DEVELOPING A COMMUNITY OF NURSES

Another group experience in which Humanistic Nursing Theory was utilized was the formation of a community of nurses who were mutually struggling with changes in their nursing roles. You will recall that the inner mandate of Humanistic Nursing Theory is to share with, thereby allowing each to become more. You will also recall that when we spoke of "call" it was indicated that the call in Humanistic Nursing Theory terms, can be from an individual, a family, a community or humanity itself. In this instance I became aware of my own experiences as a nursing care coordinator as I struggled with the changes that were happening around me and how these changes were impacting on me.

The nursing shortage, the increased salaries, even government agencies were calling for nurses to be proactive in the current health care crises. In the Secretary's Commission on Nursing (12/88) we were told, "the perspective and expertise of nurses are a necessary adjunct to that of other health care professionals in the policy-making, and regulatory, and standard setting process" (p. 31). The challenge being posed to nurses is to help create the changes in the health care system today. The ability to initiate and cause change is a definition of power (Miller, 1982, p. 2). Being asked to act and to be perceived in a powerful way was a shift for us as nurses who have historically been reactive rather than proactive. In reflecting and analyzing my own experience of this challenge I identified some anxiety about this call from the community at large. Recalling my past experience when I was anxious about trying the phenomenological method of inquiry, I identified that going through the process with a group of nurses who were experiencing the same newness was helpful. I called to the community of nurses where I work, and we joined together to struggle with this challenge. For while the importance of organized nursing power cannot be overemphasized, it is the individual nurse in her day to day practice who can actualize or undermine the power of the profession.

In settings such as hospitals the time pressure, the unending tasks, the emotional strain and the conflicts do not allow nurses to relate, reflect, and support each other in their struggle toward a center which is nursing. This isolation and alienation does not allow for the development of either a personal or professional voice. Within our community of nurses it became clear that developing individual voices was clearly our first task. Talking and listening to each other about our nursing worlds allowed us to become more articulate and clear about function and value as nurses. The theme of developing an articulate voice has pervaded and continues to pervade this group. There is an ever increasing awareness of both manner and language as we interact with each other and those outside the group. The resolve for an articulate voice is even more firm as members of the group experience and share the empowering effect it can have on both one's personal and professional life. It has been said that, "Those that express themselves unfold in health, beauty, and human potential. They become unblocked channels through which creativity can flow" (Hills & Stone, 1976, p. 71).

Group members offered alternative approaches to various situations that were utilized and subsequently brought back to the group. In this way each member shared in the experience. That experience therefore became available to all members as they individually formulated their own knowledge base and expanded their angular view. As Dr. Paterson and Dr. Zderad present, "each person might be viewed as a community of the beings with whom she has meaningfully related" (p. 45); and as a potential resource for expanding herself as a "knowing place."

Through openness and sharing we were able to differentiate our strengths. Once the members could truly appreciate the unique competence of each other they were able to reflect that appreciation back. Through this reflection members began to internalize and then project a competent image of themselves. They learned that this positive mirroring did not have to come from outsiders. They can reflect back to each other the image of competence and power. They as a community of nurses can empower each other. This reciprocity is a self-enhancing process for "the degree to which I can create relationships which facilitate the growth of others as separate persons is a measure of the growth I have achieved in myself" (Rogers, 1976, p. 79). And so by sharing in our community of nurses we can empower each other through mutual confirmation as we help each other move toward a center that is nursing. This is an example of Martin Buber's previously described but worth repeating, basic human need to be confirmed by others of their kind, "secretly and bashfully (they) watch for a "Yes" which allows (them) to be" (p. 71). We as nurses strive to do this with our patients. We as nurses must also strive to do this for each other and the profession of nursing.

THE CALL OF HUMANITY

Today I perceive another call. This call is resounded in and exemplified by the following description of examining a pregnant woman, "Instead of having to approach the woman, to rest your head near her belly, to smell her skin, to feel her breathing you could now read the information (on her and her fetus) from across the room, from down the hall" (Rothman, 1987, p. 28).

The call I hear is for nursing. It is the call from humanity to maintain the humanness in the health care system which is becoming increasingly sophisticated in technology, increasingly concerned with cost containment, and increasingly less aware of and concerned with the patient as a human being. The context of humanistic nursing theory is humans. The basic question it asks of nursing practice is, "Is this particular intersubjective-transactional nursing event humanizing or dehumanizing?" Nurses as clinicians, teachers, researchers and administrators can use the concepts and process of humanistic nursing theory to gain a better understanding of the "calls" we are hearing. Through this understanding we are given direction for expanding ourselves as "knowing places" so that we can fulfill our reason for being which, according to humanistic nursing theory, is nurturing the well-being and more-being of persons in need.

REFERENCES

Buber, M. (1965). *The knowledge of man.* New York: Harper & Row Publishers, Inc.

Hills, C., & Stone, R. B. (1976). *Conduct your own awareness sessions: 100 ways to enhance self-concept in the classroom.* New Jersey: Prentice Hall, Inc.

Miller, J. B. (1976). *Toward a new psychology of woman.* Boston: Beacon Press.

Paterson, J. G. (1977). *Living until death, my perspective.* Paper presented at the Syracuse Veteran's Administration Hospital.

Paterson, J. G., & Zderad, L. T. (1976). *Humanistic Nursing.* New York: John Wiley & Sons.

Rogers, C. R. (1976). *Perceiving, behaving, and becoming: 100 ways to enhance self-concept in the classroom.* New Jersey: Prentice Hall, Inc.

Rothman, B. (1987). *The tentative pregnancy: Prenatal diagnosis and the future of motherhood.* New York: Penguin.

U. S. Public Health Services. (12/88). *Secretary's commission on nursing, final report.* Washington, DC: Department of Health & Human Services.

Zderad, L. T. (1978). From here-and-now the theory: Reflections on "how." In *Theory development: What? why? how?* New York: National League for Nursing Press.

Part III

Parse's Human Becoming Theory

5

Parse's Human Becoming Theory: Its Research and Practice Implications

Rosemarie Rizzo Parse

The 1990s is the decade of nursing knowledge-based practice and research. This means that nurse researchers and nurse leaders in practice, education, and administration are formulating anew what they "do" to be consistent with what they "know" as the knowledge base of nursing. This knowledge base is embedded in the extant nursing theories and frameworks and continues to expand through research. The expansion of unique nursing knowledge is essential to the survival of the discipline.

The scientific discipline of nursing is a body of basic knowledge created by nurses from the time of Florence Nightingale (1859/1946). Nightingale posited three major concepts as nursing's phenomena of concern: human being, environment, and health. These concepts specified as the human-universe-health process remain the central concern of nursing today. In examining the nursing literature related to these concepts, Parse (Parse, Coyne & Smith, 1985) organized the knowledge base according to beliefs about the relationships among these three concepts. She identified two major perspectives in the nursing literature on the human-universe-health relationship. One view identifies the human being as an organism, composed of body, mind, and spirit. The human-universe relationship in this view is cause-effect in nature with humans responding to and manipulating the environment. Health from this perspective is a state of physical, mental, and spiritual well-being determined by societal norms. Disease is the opposite of health and can be prevented through manipulation of the environment. This world-view is the totality paradigm (Parse, 1987). The other perspective, the simultaneity paradigm, emerged in the early 1970s and is a growing force in nursing as the 21st century approaches. The simultaneity paradigm (Parse et al., 1985; Parse, 1987) posits the human being as unitary, recognized through pattern and mutual process with the universe. Health is viewed as a process incarnating values not dependent on societal norms. Parse's theory emerges from the simultaneity paradigm.

To understand better the flow of Parse's theory, certain definitions are helpful. A *theory* is a set of interrelated concepts written at the same level of discourse to describe, explain, or predict the phenomena of a discipline. An *assumption* is a statement about the phenomenon of concern to a discipline. It is written at the highest level of abstraction, the philosophical level of discourse, and is the set of beliefs that the theorist holds to be true. A *concept* is an abstract idea expressed in a word or phrase written at the theoretical level of discourse. It is a building block of a theory. A *principle* is a statement explaining a phenomenon by joining two or more concepts written at the theoretical level. A *proposition* is a statement relating two or more concepts from the principles to guide research and practice. Propositions are written at an empirical level of discourse. The philosophical, theoretical, and empirical levels of discourse are stated in terms that are in decreasing levels of abstraction, with the empirical being the most concrete. A theory is a description of the phenomenon of concern to a discipline (Parse, 1987, pp. 2–3).

A METAPERSPECTIVE OF PARSE'S THEORY

Parse's theory of man-living-health (Parse, 1981) has recently been renamed Parse's theory of human becoming (Parse, 1992). No aspect of the theory itself has been changed. The renaming was necessary when the English dictionary definition of the term man changed. In 1980 when the theory was written, the definition for man was *mankind*, but now the meaning is *male gender*, thus no longer reflecting Parse's intent. Parse's theory is a human science theory unlike most others. Human science refers to the human being's participative experience with the world. Human science nursing theory has its roots in the belief that humans participate with the world in the cocreation of health (Parse, 1981). This theory takes into consideration that human beings live health, a set of personal values. Each individual's own lived values are primary, and it is from the person's vantage point that the nurse enters the person's world.

The concepts are written as participles with the "ing" ending. This was deliberately designed to make explicit the process orientation of the theory. For example, *power* has a more static meaning than *powering*. The hyphens in the man-living-health title were designed to specify man-living-health as the construct central to the theory. Human becoming reflects this unity which is the focus of the theory. Thus, in the theory, there is *no* reference to particulate aspects of humans, such as biological, psychological, or spiritual.

PHILOSOPHICAL ASSUMPTIONS

The philosophical assumptions are written at the philosophical level of discourse and the principles and theoretical structures at the theoretical level, consistent with appropriate levels of abstraction for theory construction. Researchers and practitioners can lower the discourse of the theoretical structures to the empirical level. For example, *powering is a way of revealing-concealing imaging* can be lowered in discourse to *struggling toward goals discloses and withholds the significance of situations.* This empirically stated proposition means that the ups and downs lived in moving toward achieving something both tell and do not tell what is important to a person.

Parse's theory is grounded in nine assumptions, four about the human being and five about health (Parse, 1981, 1992). There are three about human becoming (Parse, in Parse et al., 1985; Parse, 1992). The theory consists of three major principles, each joining three concepts written at the same level of discourse; thus, there are nine concepts. One concept from each principle is connected in a unique way to formulate theoretical structures which can be used to guide research and practice (Parse, 1981, p. 68). Any number of combinations of concepts from each principle can be structured by researchers and practitioners to guide their work.

The philosophical assumptions of the theory are derived from ideas from Rogers' framework and tenets from existential phenomenology (Parse, 1981, 1992). Four assumptions (Parse, 1981, 1992) specify the human as an open being in mutual process with the universe, cocreating patterns of relating. The human lives at multidimensional realms of the universe all at once, freely choosing ways of becoming as meaning is given to situations. The possibles are the cherished hopes and dreams that a person is incarnating with his or her life.

The other five assumptions specify health as becoming, coconstituted through the human-universe mutual process, and incarnated as patterns of relating value priorities (Parse, 1981, 1992). Becoming is an intersubjective transcending with possibles in the process of unfolding. Each assumption is a synthesis of concepts juxtaposed in such a way as to create the underpinnings of a new product, Parse's theory of human becoming (Parse, 1981, 1992). A detailed discussion of the original assumptions can be found in Parse, 1981, pp. 23–36. The updated version specified in terms of human becoming can be found in Parse, 1992, pp. 35–42.

These assumptions express in philosophical terms the beliefs that underpin the theory of human becoming. The most significant distinction of this theory which specifies it as different from other theories is the belief that the human is unitary, evolves mutually with the universe, participates in cocreating personal health by freely choosing meaning in situations, and conveys meanings that are personal values incarnating dreams and hopes. These beliefs represent a very different view of the human than that posited by other theories and frameworks. The human becoming theory is clearly distinct from totality paradigm theories and frameworks as reflected in the definition of the human being, the nature of the human-universe process, and the meaning of health. While Parse drew on Rogers' framework in constructing the human becoming theory, it is distinct from Rogerian science. Rogerian science specifies the human as an energy field recognized by field pattern, while Parse describes the human as an open being cocreating becoming with the universe recognized through paradoxical patterns of relating and freely choosing in situations. Health for Rogers is a value, and for Parse it is one's personal path or way of becoming.

PRINCIPLES OF PARSE'S THEORY

Three major themes arise from these philosophical assumptions, *meaning, rhythmicity and cotranscendence*. Each is specified in a principle of Parse's theory of human becoming. The principles are written at the theoretical level of discourse. There are nine major concepts in the theory, three explaining each of the principles. The concepts from principle 1 are imaging, valuing, languaging; from principle 2 revealing-concealing, enabling-limiting, connecting-separating; from principle 3 powering, originating, and transforming. The principles of Parse's human becoming theory incarnate the beliefs articulated in the assumptions and can be found in Parse, 1981, pp. 37–75, and Parse, 1992, pp. 37–39.

The theory as specified in these principles explicates paradox as fundamental to the human-universe process. Paradox refers to apparent opposites but is really one rhythm with two co-existent distinguishable dimensions. Humans live paradoxical rhythms of relating with the universe. The paradoxes are not phenomena to be resolved or individual inconsistencies but rather are ways humans live meaning. In human unfolding there is always the mystery of ambiguity which gives rise to the paradoxical movement. Paradox is present in all of the principles but most explicit in principle 2.

The first principle explicates the idea that humans construct meaning from various realms of the universe, the tacit-explicit, in cocreating reality. Reality, personally structured meaning, is the incarnation of one's value priorities represented through symbols disclosed in moving and speaking. The paradoxes present in principle 1 are: *tacit-explicit* knowing, which refers to the *prereflective-reflective* process of imaging the real; *confirming-disconfirming*, which refers to choosing and changing in the process of valuing; and *speaking – being silent* and *moving – being still*, which refer to the symbols of languaging.

The second principle describes the rhythmical patterns of relating with the universe as paradoxical unities. The concept *revealing-concealing* describes the simultaneous withholding-disclosing in human relationships. One cannot withhold or disclose all there is about self to self or others. Not all is known explicitly in the unfolding mystery of human becoming. *Enabling-limiting* refers to the opportunities and limitations simultaneously present in choosing to move in one direction while giving up others. *Connecting-separating* is the rhythmical process of coming together with and moving apart from phenomena. In coming together there is the closeness of togetherness and the distance of moving apart from the same phenomenon, and in moving apart there is both distance and closeness all at once. The paradoxical movement is a rhythmical cadence ever more diverse in the ebb and flow of life.

The third principle specifies that humans are continuously changing in moving beyond the moment to the not-yet. The changing unfolds as experience melts into experience and the fabric of meaning becomes more diverse. The paradoxical rhythm of *pushing-resisting* is the energizing force of powering in the human-universe process. The forging-ahead – holding-back is a cadent movement in the natural order-disorder of life, as humans create new ways of becoming through living the *conformity – non-conformity* of originating. Humans seek to be like others and not like others all at once. Choices to conform – not conform are made in light of the *certainty-uncertainty* embedded in all change. The changing is with the *familiar-unfamiliar* of transforming. The transformation unfolds as the familiar is viewed in a new and unfamiliar light. The realm of the familiar is also already laden with what is not known, just as the unfamiliar is penetrated by what is already known.

The three principles set forth the essence of the theory by making explicit the nature of the human-universe-health process. Theoretical structures link the theory to research and practice.

THEORETICAL STRUCTURES

The theoretical structures of Parse's human becoming theory are non-directional propositions. They are non-causal in nature and consistent with the assumptions and principles of the theory. Theoretical structures are written at the theoretical level and are designed to guide research and practice. In creating the structures it is appropriate to use one concept from each principle to preserve the integrity of the theory as a description of the human-universe-health process. In order for these to become operational in research and practice, propositions at a lower level of discourse must be derived and lived experiences chosen for study. (See Parse, 1981, pp. 77–90, for examples in research and practice.) Examples of theoretical structures are:

1. Powering is a way of revealing-concealing imaging.

2. Originating is a manifestation of enabling-limiting valuing.

3. Transforming unfolds in the languaging of connecting-separating (Parse, 1981, p. 72).

RESEARCH AND PRACTICE TRADITIONS IN NURSING

Thus far, the research and practice methodologies utilized in the discipline of nursing have been mostly borrowed from other disciplines.

Nursing is just beginning to develop its own research methodologies (Parse, 1987, 1990a, 1990b). In 1987, Parse developed research and practice methodologies congruent with the human becoming theory, and with this development a unique research tradition for nursing was born. The Parse theory is the only one to have both a research and practice tradition including the ontology with congruent research and practice methodologies.

Parse's Practice Methodology

Parse's practice methodology has three major dimensions which are discussed in detail in Parse, 1987, pp. 168–171; Parse, 1990a, pp. 136–140; and Parse, 1992, pp. 39–42. These dimensions are: illuminating meaning, synchronizing rhythms, and mobilizing transcendence (Parse, 1987, p. 67). *Illuminating meaning* involves the nurse in true presence inviting persons to relate the meaning of situations. In telling about the meaning, persons share thoughts and feelings with the nurse, and in a nurse-family situation, with one another. This process in itself sheds a different light on the situation for the person. The sharing of meaning is not so the nurse can gather information but rather so the person has an opportunity to articulate explicitly in his or her own words how the situation is viewed. *Synchronizing rhythms* is lived as the person in the true presence of the nurse describes the meaning of the moment, the struggles, moments of joy, and the unevenness of day-to-day living. The nurse practicing from the human becoming theory does not try to calm uneven rhythms but, rather, goes with the rhythms set by the person or family. The nurse in true presence moves with the flow of the rhythm as the person or family discusses and recognizes the harmony within the struggles of the situation (Parse, 1992). *Mobilizing transcendence* happens in true presence with the nurse as individuals and families move beyond the moment, planning to reach the hopes and dreams that have been illuminated through the nurse-person process.

The specific processes inherent in the dimensions are defined as follows:

Explicating is a process of making clear what is appearing now through languaging.

Dwelling with is giving self over to the flow of the struggle in connecting-separating.

Moving beyond is propelling toward the possibles in transforming (Parse, 1987, p. 167).

These dimensions and processes are lived all at once with the nurse in true presence with the person or family. They are not serial steps or activities as specified in the well-known nursing process.

Nursing practice from Parse's perspective is different from the traditional practice of nursing. It is "not offering professional advice and opinions stemming from the nurse's own lived value system. It is not a canned approach to care. It is a subject-to-subject interrelationship, a loving true presence with the other to enhance the quality of life" (Parse, 1987, p. 169). True presence is a non-routinized, non-mechanical way of "being with" in which the nurse is attentive to moment-to-moment changes in meaning for the person or group. True presence is cocreated as an intentional reflective love which the nurse shares with the other as the other and the nurse blossom according to personal desires and dreams. "Intentional reflective love is an interpersonal art grounded in a strong knowledge base reflecting the belief that each person knows the way somewhere within self. Each person lives a way, his or her *own* way, which is both alike and different from the ways of others. It is *like* that of others in that it is a personal way of being; each individual has a personal way of being. It is *different* from others in that it is one's own. It is like a fingerprint in that it belongs to only one human being and while others coexist in the large journey of life, each lives his or her own way on the journey" (Parse, 1990a, p. 139).

Living a true presence with the person or family is placing the emphasis on the human-to-human interrelationship, with the nurse valuing the person as co-author freely choosing personal health. "The nurse in true presence is not a guide or a beacon with the person and family, but rather an inspiring attentive presence that calls the other to shed light on the meaning moments of his or her life. It is the person in the presence of the nurse that illuminates the meaning, synchronizes the rhythms, and mobilizes transcendence in moving beyond. The person is coauthor of health, free agent, and meaning giver, choosing rhythmical patterns of relating while reaching for personal hopes and dreams" (Parse, 1992, p. 40).

True presence is a powerful interhuman connection experienced at all realms of one's universe. What happens in the immediate moment of coming together lingers as each person moves on to different situations. The *lingering presence* is a haunting reflective-prereflective "abiding with" attended to through glimpses of the other person, idea, object, or situation. These glimpses know no boundaries. They arise in and out of similar contexts—moments, days, or years later, and they can be startling surprises, calming excursions, or uncomfortable intrusions. The lingering presence of another may not even surface as a recognizable glimpse of a particular experience or at all. An experience of true presence is weaved somehow into the fabric of one's life through this lingering presence. For nursing practice, this means that in true presence with another all of the realms of the universe of the nurse and the person are interconnecting, reflectively and pre-reflectively; thus, *how* the nurse *is with* the person is extremely important—multiple messages are both given and taken. The intent of the nurse's "being with" is felt and disclosed at many realms even when it is explicitly withheld from the other.

The goal in Parse practice is the quality of life as described by the person and the family (Parse, 1981). The context where nursing arises is in nurse-person or nurse-group situations. Several nurse-person situations utilizing Parse's practice methodology have been published. Butler (1988) told a dramatic story of a Parse nurse present with a family during the father's hospitalization and discharge. Mitchell (1988) described true presence in practice with a woman who moved from an acute care setting through three months on a rehabilitation unit with discharge to a home for the aged. Liehr (1989) described the meaning of true presence in another nurse-person situation. Mitchell and Pilkington (1990) compared the theory-based approaches of Parse and Roy in the care of a particular person, pointing out many differences related to the theories and the goals of nursing. Mitchell (1990a) described the struggle that she encountered in moving from a traditional nursing approach to the practice of Parse's theory. She discussed in detail the meaning of changing beliefs about human beings and health and the inner struggle in developing expertise in the practice of Parse's theory. These are just a few examples of published work on Parse's theory in practice; several other articles appear in journals in the United States, Canada, and Japan.

Parse's Research Methodology

Research related to Parse's theory has been and continues to be implemented using the phenomenological, ethnographic, and descriptive methods. These methods, though borrowed, are consistent with the ontology of the human becoming theory. In 1987, Parse (1987) invented a new research methodology. In construction of the research methodology for the human becoming theory, three major essentials were considered: the basic assumptions of the theory, the principles of the theory, and the principles of method construction. Details of the method construction appear in Parse, 1987, pp. 172–180.

A research tradition includes both ontological and methodological elements. The ontology is the belief system about the phenomenon of concern to the discipline. The methodology is the approach to inquiry. The methodology derived from Parse's theory includes identification of major entities for study and scientific processes for investigation. (See Parse, 1987, p. 173, for details.)

Entities for Study. The major entities to be considered for inquiry with Parse's research method are universal human experiences. A universal human experience is one that persons of all ages could describe, for example, grieving, hope, and suffering. Research questions appropriate when using Parse's methodology are: What is the structure of the lived experience of joy? What is the structure of the lived experience of suffering? Experiences are lived in multidimensional universes all at once. An understanding of the entity can be gained through the processes of the method. The purpose of the method is to uncover the structure as lived by the participant. The structure is the paradoxical living of the remembered, the now moment, and the not-yet all at once (Parse, 1987). This structure is uncovered through the dialogical engagement between the researcher and participant, as the participant describes in detail the meaning of the lived experience under study in the true presence of the researcher.

Processes of the Method. The processes of the method include participant selection, dialogical engagement, extraction-synthesis, and heuristic interpretation. Participants are persons able to describe living the experience. An assumption is that a person who agrees to participate in a study about a particular lived experience can share a description of that experience when engaged in dialogue with the researcher. Participants may draw pictures or use poetry, metaphors, or other symbols to describe the experience, but these are interpreted by the persons themselves in telling the stories of their meanings (Parse, 1992). Redundancy is sought in determining adequacy in number of participants.

Dialogical engagement is the researcher-participant discussion. The researcher in true presence with the participant moves through an unstructured discussion about the lived experience. The researcher is truly present with the participant in discussion as the remembered, the now, and the not-yet unfold all at once. The intent of true presence is different in practice and research. True presence in both research and practice is an intense attentiveness, but the goal of practice is quality of life. The intent of the Parse nurse in practice is being with the person as the person unfolds personal patterns of health. The researcher's intent is to uncover essences of universal experiences to add to the knowledge base of nursing. True presence in the research method is not an interview but an "abiding with" the participant as the remembered, the now moment, and the not-yet surface the structure of the lived experience. The discussion is tape-recorded (audio and video), and the dialogue is transcribed to typed format for easy reading in the extraction-synthesis process.

Extraction-synthesis occurs through dwelling with the transcribed researcher-participant dialogue and the videotape. "Dwelling with" is a way of centering self with the descriptions. The researcher carefully contemplates the descriptions, listens to the tapes, and watches the videotapes in order to uncover the meaning of the experience for the participants. "Dwelling with" permeates the entire extraction-synthesis process.

There are five major processes in extraction-synthesis which are explained in detail in Parse, 1987, p. 187, and Parse, 1990a. Briefly they are:

1. Extracting essences from transcribed descriptions (participant's language). An extracted essence is a complete expression of a core idea described by the participant.

2. Synthesizing essences (researcher's language). A synthesized essence is an expression of the core ideas of the extracted essence conceptualized by the researcher.

3. Formulating a proposition from each participant's description. A proposition is a nondirectional statement conceptualized by the researcher joining the core ideas of the synthesized essences from each participant.

4. Extracting core concepts from the formulated propositions of all participants. An extracted core concept is the idea that captures the central meaning of the proposition.

5. Synthesizing a structure of the lived experience from the extracted core concepts. A synthesized structure is a statement conceptualized by the researcher joining the core concepts. The structure as evolved answers the research question, what is the structure of this lived experience? (Parse, 1987, p. 177)

Heuristic interpretation includes structural integration and conceptual interpretation and is the process of connecting the proposition and the structure to the concepts of Parse's theory and beyond to posit ideas for further research and practice. (See Parse, 1990b, for illustration.)

This emerging methodology differs from all other methods. It differs from those in the totality paradigm in that those methods call for a focus on linear causality in the human-universe interrelationship. The ontology of the totality paradigm leads to methods of inquiry that seek understanding of cause-effect and associative relationships among variables in order to make predictions. Parse's research methodology is also different from other qualitative methods. The unique aspects of Parse's methodology are within the dialogical engagement and the way the findings are weaved into the theory and beyond. The dialogical engagement as described above is a unique way of "being with" the participant and is not specified as part of any other qualitative research methodology. The other uniqueness is that findings of the study are taken up to the theory level and weaved together with specific concepts of the human becoming theory, as well as projecting implications for practice and further research. There are a number of published reports of research using Parse's method (Cody, 1991; Kelley, 1991; Mitchell, 1990b; Parse, 1990b; Pilkington, in press; Smith, 1990).

The human becoming theory is a unique human science theory with congruent practice and research methodologies. This ontologic-methodologic package provides the discipline with a research and practice tradition upon which to continue to build the knowledge base of nursing.

REFERENCES

Butler, M. J. (1988). Family transformation: Parse's theory in practice. *Nursing Science Quarterly*, 1, 68–74.

Cody, W. K. (1991). Grieving a personal loss. *Nursing Science Quarterly*, 4, 61–68.

Kelley, L. S. (1991). Struggling with going along when you do not believe. *Nursing Science Quarterly, 4,* 123–129.

Liehr, P. R. (1989). The core of true presence: A loving center. *Nursing Science Quarterly, 2,* 7–8.

Mitchell, G. J. (1988). Man-living-health: The theory in practice. *Nursing Science Quarterly, 1,* 120–127.

Mitchell, G. J. (1990a). Struggling in change: From the traditional approach to Parse's theory-based practice. *Nursing Science Quarterly, 3,* 170–176.

Mitchell, G. J. (1990b). The lived experience of taking life day by day in later life: Research guided by Parse's emergent method. *Nursing Science Quarterly, 3,* 29–36.

Mitchell, G. J., & Pilkington, B. (1990). Theoretical approaches in nursing practice: A comparison of Parse and Roy. *Nursing Science Quarterly, 3,* 81–87.

Nightingale, F. (1946). *Notes on nursing: What it is and what it is not.* Philadelphia: Lippincott. (Original work published 1859)

Parse, R. R. (1981). *Man-living-health: A theory of nursing.* New York: Wiley.

Parse, R. R. (1987). *Nursing science: Major paradigms, theories, and critiques.* Philadelphia: Saunders.

Parse, R. R. (1990a). Health: A personal commitment. *Nursing Science Quarterly, 3,* 136–140.

Parse, R. R. (1990b). Parse's research methodology with an illustration of the lived experience of hope. *Nursing Science Quarterly, 3,* 9–17.

Parse, R. R. (1992). Human becoming: Parse's theory of nursing. *Nursing Science Quarterly, 5,* 35–42.

Parse, R. R., Coyne, A. B., & Smith, M. J. (1985). *Nursing research: Qualitative methods.* Bowie, MD: Brady.

Pilkington, F. B. (in press). The lived experience of grieving the loss of an important other. *Nursing Science Quarterly.*

Smith, M. C. (1990). Struggling through a difficult time for unemployed persons. *Nursing Science Quarterly, 3,* 18–28.

6

Parse's Theory in Practice

Gail J. Mitchell

Parse's (1981, 1987, 1990a, 1992a) theory of human becoming offers a distinct guide for practice with all human beings, but unlike some others, this theory cannot be *applied* in the strict sense of the word. According to Webster's dictionary, the word application means to use, administer, or superimpose. The image conjured up by these terms is one of a nursing theory that is separate from the nurse, and in its separateness the theory gets picked up, used, and set down again like a pencil or a book. Parse's theory cannot be used in this fashion.

The Parse way of practice is underpinned by a distinct set of values and beliefs that nurses learn to *live* in relationship with others. To live something, according to Webster's, is to cohabit, to practice, and to be in accordance with. The image conjured by the word live is one of togetherness, consistency, and commitment. In order to practice in accordance with the beliefs of Parse's theory, a nurse must commit to learn and integrate the beliefs set forth in the assumptions, principles, and concepts.

The study of Parse's theory changes the nurse's way of thinking and acting, rather than changing the thoughts and actions of those receiving care. It will become clear that it is not Parse's theory that works or fails in practice, as some suggest, depending on the different aspects of persons and their situations. Rather, it is whether the nurse can live the values and beliefs of the theory with all persons, or not. There is a shift for nurses guided by Parse's theory of human becoming from telling, advising, managing, and controlling, to being with, participating, clarifying, and exploring. There are no interventions to apply or directives to prescribe because the persons involved with the nurse define and direct the way their health is lived.

Health is defined by persons themselves and relates to the day to day living of what is important, with those who are cherished and those who are not, according to personal values, concerns, and desires. Further, health is coconstituted with others who participate in making life what it is for every person. In Parse's theory persons are the experts when it comes to human becoming and they disclose their health in the practice relationship. Practice with Parse's theory is a living, cocreated process that unfolds in relationship with others. The nurse is called upon to live true presence, a presence that honors the other just for being human, a presence that makes a difference to the others' quality of living health (Parse, 1981, 1992a).

THE PURPOSE OF THEORY-BASED PRACTICE

Prior to considering Parse's theory in practice, it is helpful to reconsider the purpose of theory-based practice. Parse (1987) suggests that the knowledge of a discipline is housed in its theories, and different theories flow from different paradigms. The discipline of nursing has at least two paradigms that spawn theories (Parse, 1987). Further, each paradigm has different traditions of knowledge. The knowledge housed in a guiding theory shapes the way the professional thinks and acts with clients. This is important because thoughts guide actions, and actions weave relationships, and relationships form the fabric of nursing practice.

The purpose then of theory-based practice is to provide a guide for thinking and acting. Well developed theories, such as Parse's, provide a set of assumptions, principles, and concepts that are consistent with each other, and that together provide a coherent view of reality for nurses in practice and research. A nursing theory provides a filter, a kind of lens, that focuses on some phenomenon of concern to the discipline. In nursing, the phenomenon of concern has been broadly defined as the human-health interrelationship. Different theories specify unique views of the human-health interrelationship in order to provide a framework for understanding and interpreting the nursing world. For Parse, the view of the human-health interrelationship focuses on persons' ways of structuring meaning, their rhythmical patterns of relating, and their ways of cotranscending with the possibles in the living of health. The theory of human becoming is rooted in a tradition of knowledge, the human science tradition, that is concerned with the lived experiences of human beings (Parse, 1981). Dilthey (1976) suggested that the human sciences should focus on the interrelationships among life, expression, and understanding. Parse's theory adheres to this basic belief espoused by Dilthey, and further extends knowledge in unique ways for nursing science (Mitchell & Cody, 1992).

Parse's theory specifies knowledge for thinking about human experience. For example, Parse suggests that human becoming is inherently paradoxical and that no life experience is entirely black or white. Persons make decisions and move on in life by thinking about and struggling with both sides of paradoxical rhythms. For instance, a person may want to return to school in order to advance at work, and yet, not want to return because of the cost and potential disruption of family life. Or an elderly woman may want to live with an adult son, while, at the same time, wanting to live in a nursing home in order to avoid being a burden to the child. Both of these individuals struggle with the possible consequences of moving in any one direction. Both speak of possible benefits and potential restrictions as they consider different aspects of their paradoxical thoughts and feelings. The nurse guided by Parse's theory understands paradoxical struggles and is guided to go with the person/family as different aspects of the rhythm are explored. The struggle and movement between wanting one thing, while at the same time wanting another, is viewed as an aspect of the person's becoming as value priorities shift in life. The nurse practicing with Parse's theory respects the paradoxical rhythm, bears witness to the other's inherent struggle in moving beyond, and lives true presence as the person/family structures the meaning of changing situations.

The reason a nurse guided by Parse's theory understands paradoxical rhythms as an inherent aspect of lived experience is because of the knowledge base of the human becoming theory. Nurses practicing with traditional bio-psycho-social theories may recognize the opposing sides of a paradoxical rhythm, or they may not. If recognized, paradox is typically labelled in traditional theories as ambivalence, a term with negative connotations, a problem to be fixed. Additionally, borrowed bio-psycho-social theories guide nurses to try to eliminate ambivalence by giving advice or directives that are based on norms and predefined standards. Parse proposes that the person is the expert and knows the best decisions to make in life. Whether or not the woman described above should return to school, or whether the elderly individual should move in with her son or go to a nursing home, are decisions to be made by the persons themselves rather than outsiders. No one, not even the persons themselves, can know all the consequences of their decisions and Parse guides the nurse to see all choices as both enabling and limiting. With every decision some doors open and others close as persons move and become their unique selves. In Parse's theory, persons make choices based on what is important to them, and they also bear responsibility for the consequences of personal decisions (Parse, 1990a, 1992a).

The purpose of theory-based practice is to guide the nurse's participation with persons according to a scientific knowledge base in a consistent way toward clearly defined goals. In Parse's theory the knowledge is rooted in the simultaneity paradigm, a belief system with specific philosophical assumptions, that anchors Parse's substantive content about meanings, rhythms, and transcendence as specified in the principles and concepts. The theory is a coherent whole that guides nurses' thoughts and actions in practice and research. The goal of Parse's theory is quality of life as defined by persons themselves.

LEARNING TO LIVE PARSE'S THEORY

Learning about Parse's theory involves a process of reflecting, integrating, and changing. Reflection is a process of deliberately considering and questioning some thought or idea. Parse's theory is complex and multilayered. Nurses are encouraged to think about and question the assumptions and beliefs outlined in the human becoming theory. For instance, when first considering Parse's theory a nurse may explore whether the notion of unitary human being—a living unity more than and different from the sum of parts—is a belief that can be embraced. If a nurse concludes that the notion of unitary is appealing and consistent with personal beliefs and experience then the theory might be further explored. But it is one thing to embrace a belief in a moment of reflection and another to then integrate and commit to live that belief in practice and research activities. This is because most nurses have only been educated with traditional theoretical knowledge that fragments human beings into their biological, psychological, social, spiritual, cultural parts.

For example, a nurse may endorse the belief that human beings are unitary or irreducible to their bio-psycho-social parts. The very next day this same nurse may be with a person who speaks of not wanting to think about the death of a loved one because it is too painful and because by pretending the death is not real, the pain is less. Because of an already established knowledge base, the nurse begins to judge the person's experience as denial, a psychological defense mechanism used to avoid reality. This psychological label is not consistent with the unitary view of persons. Interventions aimed at changing the person's reality may automatically come to mind. Nurses living Parse's theory do not believe in causal interventions that aim to change the other's reality. The nurse's former knowledge base is still there even though the unitary perspective was embraced at some level.

Further, there is no judging or labelling in practice guided by Parse's theory. The very process of setting others apart and comparing their thoughts and actions to some standard of normal is antithetical to the basic beliefs and value of Parse's theory (Mitchell, 1991). From Parse's perspective, the person who speaks of not thinking about the death of a loved one does not need to be fixed or moved to a different reality. Research guided by Parse's theory has shed light on how persons grieving the loss of another live a rhythm of connecting-separating with the absent presence and others (Cody, 1991; Pilkington, in press). Not thinking of the one who has died is a way of connecting-separating with the one who has gone as well as the pain of loss, and the person knows best how to live the connecting-separating rhythm. Until the nurse's new beliefs become integrated and show themselves in practice, Parse's theory is not being lived.

The nurse learning Parse's theory restructures former beliefs in order to facilitate the growth of a new knowledge base, a knowledge base that redefines the nurse's way of looking at the human-universe-health interrelationship. So even though a nurse may embrace a unitary view of human beings, for example, there is a time required before the belief can be lived in practice. The time may be several weeks, or months before the shift from one knowledge base, one scientific tradition, to another is integrated. Learning Parse's theory is challenging and at times frustrating. In integrating the knowledge base of Parse's theory, there is a rhythm of clarity-obscurity described by many nurses. This paradoxical rhythm represents the sudden glimpses of new insight and understanding that occur in the sea of obscurity when engaging a whole new way of thinking. In order to grow and learn with the theory, the nurse needs to be committed, open, and willing to live with risk and uncertainty. This can be especially difficult given nursing's recent history of depending on policies and procedures, assessment tools, and the linear nursing process for defining practice. Jourard (1972) suggests that each human being embodies personal commitments. In other words, commitments are lived in human actions, and as new commitments are made throughout life there is a change in values and a change in the way a person lives. Learning Parse's theory requires such a commitment, a commitment to live a different way in the nurse-person relationship.

The new knowledge base of the human becoming theory is grown in layers through the careful study of Parse's (1981, 1987, 1990a, 1990b, 1992a, 1992b) work and that of those who are guided by her theory in research and practice. Published articles related to practice describe health and human becoming for persons and families in various situations (Butler, 1988; Butler & Snodgrass, 1991; Mattice & Mitchell, 1990; Mitchell, 1986, 1988; Mitchell & Copplestone, 1990; Mitchell & Pilkington, 1990; Mitchell & Santopinto, 1988; Rasmusson, Jonas, & Mitchell, 1991). Researchers have explored lived experiences like recovering from addiction (Banonis, 1989), grieving (Cody, 1991, 1992; Pilkington, in press), being an elder (Jonas, 1992), struggling with going along when you do not believe (Kelley, 1991), taking life day-by-day (Mitchell, 1990a), restriction-freedom in later life (Mitchell, 1992), living with AIDS (Nokes & Carver, 1991), hope (Parse, 1990b), the relentless drive to be ever thinner (Santopinto, 1989), struggling through a difficult time (Smith, 1990) and aging and health in the oldest-old (Wondolowski & Davis, 1988; 1991). Nurses have written about their personal experiences of learning Parse's theory, and they have specified the ways the theory changed practice and views of nursing (Mattice, 1991; Mitchell, 1990b; Quiquero, Knights, & Meo, 1991). Parse's theory of human becoming has been evaluated (Cody & Mitchell, 1992; Cowling, 1989; Phillips, 1987; Smith & Heudopohl, 1990) and explored in light of philosophical underpinnings (Mitchell & Cody, 1992; Nagle & Mitchell, 1991; Smith, 1991). There are also many non-nursing works that contribute knowledge about the human science tradition and unitary human beings (see for example, Dilthey, 1976, 1977; Ermarth, 1983; Giorgi, 1970, 1985; Heidegger, 1962; Kockelmans, 1985; Polkinghorne, 1983).

The practice of Parse's theory requires a commitment to *live* a certain set of values and beliefs, rather than to *apply* something separate. Nurses will notice when learning Parse's theory that persons in practice and research do not fracture or reduce themselves into bio-psycho-social-spiritual-cultural parts. Persons speak of their experiences in a unitary way by using phrases like, "I think I'm going to go ahead," "I feel frightened about it," "I want to see if I can do it on my own," and "I know my family will be okay." Further, the notion of mutual process, an essential aspect of the simultaneity paradigm, conceptualizes the person as a unity who both changes and is changed by the environment in such a way that neither can be considered as separate. From this simultaneity perspective the person-environment are intertwined, and any mention of person or family always means person/family in relation to complex, multidimensional worlds of meaning, relationships, culture, history, and language.

Parse (1981) describes the person as a living unity in the world who relates with the universe at many different realms. Thus, there is no subjective-objective duality in Parse's theory. Indeed, the words subjective-objective do not have meaning in the human science tradition envisioned by Dilthey (1976, 1977) and extended by Parse. The nurse's focus on unitary human beings and their lived experiences will surface many opportunities to be with persons as they describe themselves in their own realities. The nurse guided by Parse's theory in practice does not translate lived experience into diagnostic labels or other biomedical terms. Rather, the nurse stays with persons, and uses language spoken in everyday living, in the persons' own words for recording personal health descriptions, nurse-person actions, and hopes and dreams.

PARSE'S PRACTICE METHOD

Parse's practice dimensions and processes are: "illuminating meaning through explicating, synchronizing rhythms through dwelling with, and mobilizing transcendence through moving beyond" (1987, p. 167). The practice method flows from Parse's principles and links to the three themes, meaning, rhythmicity, and transcendence. The practice dimensions and processes describe what happens when the nurse is truly present with others (for a more thorough description of the practice method see Parse, 1987, 1990a, 1992a).

Prior to being present with another, the nurse centers self in order to focus with intent on the other's becoming. Parse (1992b) posits that the centering of true presence is an intentional process of emptying self in order to become full with the other's presence. Nurses may center themselves through imaging or through a process of reflecting about the person in light of Parse's principles. Parse offers questions that may be used by the nurse to center on the person/family. For example, what is most important to you right now? and what are your hopes and dreams? It is important to note that the questions are not meant to be asked in interview style. Rather, the nurse considers the questions in light of the human becoming knowledge base and then goes with the persons' descriptions and expressions. The nurse's intent is to journey with the person/family, to bear witness to their living health as it unfolds in the meanings, rhythms, and ways of moving beyond. True presence is an intentional way of "being with" that honors the other's intersubjective relationship with the world. Persons, in the true presence of the nurse, disclose, unveil, discover, relate, and transcend. Through these experiences, the person's health changes and the nurse's practice is realized. All this happens without any intent on the nurse's part to predefine or direct those changes. Rather, the nurse commits to live true presence, and this commitment, this choice is a way of coparticipating with others as they coauthor their health and quality of life.

When persons speak about the meaning of their personal situations in the nurse's true presence several things happen or surface in the nurse-person relationship. First, Parse suggests that when persons speak about the meaning of their personal situations the meaning changes. Meaning is changed when it is made explicit through spoken or written words. Persons describe this change of meaning in practice. For example, an elderly man spoke about feeling low when others looked at him like he was crazy. He said he did not even know that he felt that way until he said it out loud. The low feeling "had been lurking in his mind," he said, and when the nurse was with him, "it came out." Other persons in practice have said things like, "I didn't know I felt that way"; or "It surprises me I said that, but I do think that way"; and "Now that I've said that, I'm glad it's out." Something happens when words are formed, in the choosing of the meaning, and the tone and cadence of speaking. Persons see things in a new light when they are with the nurse and the light illuminates meaning.

A second happening that surfaces in the nurse's true presence is that as meaning is illuminated there is a synchronizing of rhythms. The synchronizing of rhythms is witnessed as persons dwell with questions, alternatives, paradoxical feelings, fears, hopes, and dreams. Parse guides nurses to go with persons as they shift their rhythms, moving from one place to another as choices are considered and consequences anticipated. It is not unusual to hear persons say that the nurse guided by Parse's theory made a difference because there was no attempt to control thoughts or feelings. Even when persons knew their thoughts did not make sense, or when the ideas were really not serious, there was a purpose in saying them. To speak words is a way of moving beyond, according to Parse. This is consistent with the belief that ideas and thoughts themselves are expansions of self (Grudin, 1990). Parse posits that illuminating meaning and synchronizing rhythms are ways of moving beyond, which is also an expanding of self.

For instance, Mrs. M was told she had a cancer that was inoperable. She immediately started thinking of all the terrible things that were going to happen to her and she wondered if life was worth living at all. As she considered getting sick, having pain, losing her hair, facing death, and even taking her own life, the nurse guided by Parse's theory went with her without trying to reassure her fears, or teach her about the stages of grieving, or about other available treatment options. When persons' experiences are compared to standards or normal stages, their humanity and dignity are trivialized. In the true presence of the Parse nurse the woman found her own place of comfort with how to be with her illness, without being judged or restrained. When this woman stopped talking about all the possibles, she thanked the nurse for just letting her say all those things. She said, "I know I'm not going to kill myself or anything, but I had to think about it. Maybe it gave me a chance to decide to live." As this meaning came to light in the lull of shifting rhythms Mrs. M was cotranscending with the possibles in the true presence of the nurse.

Parse proposes that human beings are continuously changing and becoming. This process of ongoing change represents a moving beyond the now moment. Persons move beyond in the true presence of the nurse by discovering insights about themselves and their relationships, by engaging fears and concerns, and by thinking about and making plans to live hopes and dreams. The nurse does not attempt to direct the other's way of moving beyond because the person is the one who knows the way. Choosing that way, finding out about it, what it means, and how to move along life's path, is what persons discover for themselves when nurses live true presence. And the nurse, filled with the other's presence, learns about life and about how others structure meaning, and live their chosen values, relationships, fears, hopes, and dreams. The practice dimensions and processes happen all at once as nurses co-participate in the other's creation of health and quality of life.

Parse's Theory in Hospital-Based Practice

Mr. P was a television producer when he experienced two cerebrovascular accidents within one month of each other. The first stroke left him paralyzed on the right and unable to speak; the second stroke immobilized his left side. Mr. P was considered a paraplegic with little hope of recovery. He did begin to speak and after six months was transferred to a rehabilitation hospital. Nurses working with Mr. P at the rehabilitation hospital were guided by Parse's theory of nursing. On admission, they recorded the following health description as described by Mr. P.

Personal Health Description. Mr. P says he is excited about having rehabilitation because he believes he will walk again, and when he walks again, his wife will come back to him. He says life has been a terrible ordeal and he feels down most of the time. When asked what the ordeal has been like, Mr. P said he feels trapped in a prison that is far worse than metal bars. He sees a darkness and says his pain is unbearable at times. Mr. P said he does not know how to get out of his prison but he knows he will be out if he gets to walk. He thinks he needs a plan to find some way to live on until he can get out. The only thing that has helped Mr. P so far is making pictures in his mind. He says he paints pictures of pain, and he hopes someday to be able to draw his prison. Although down deep he does not think he will ever walk, Mr. P says he still has hope even though he can't see it most days.

Mr. P's Plans, Hopes, and Dreams.

1. Mr. P plans to go to therapy twice a day to work on gaining strength.

2. Mr. P plans to contact his wife to see if she will come visit him.

3. Mr. P hopes that he will be able to paint pictures of his pain.

4. Mr. P hopes to start walking and to return to work.

Nurses guided by Parse's theory record the personal health descriptions of individuals and families in practice. On a daily basis charting includes the person's progress toward plans and hopes as described and evaluated by the *person*. For example, a nurse charted that Mr. P said he is not gaining as much strength as he hoped but that his arms are moving a bit. Although he has not called his wife yet, he does plan to call her soon. Mr. P said he still feels down but that it helps to talk about the pain. All descriptions recorded by the nurse represent the person's meanings, concerns, and thoughts about what is happening, as well as their plans for moving toward what is wanted.

In discussions with the nurse, persons disclose paradoxical patterns that can guide further nurse-person actions over time. Mr. P described two paradoxical patterns of becoming as indicated in the following.

Patterns of Becoming	Nurse-Person Actions
Mr. P says he is excited about having rehabilitation and that he is hopeful, yet he feels trapped in a prison of darkness and pain.	Clarify what Mr. P hopes to achieve with rehabilitation and what he can do to move toward those hopes. Explore Mr. P's thoughts about his prison and feelings of being trapped. Explore his desire to paint pictures of his pain and ask him to describe details of what the pain looks like.
Mr. P believes he will walk again, yet he thinks he will not make it.	Ask Mr. P if he can picture himself walking and what it is like. Explore what he can do to move toward his dream. Ask him what he meant by not making it and what that will be like.

Mr. P continues to live in a chronic care setting. He was not walking after six months but he still had hope. Mr. P did begin to draw and paint pictures with the movement that returned to one of his arms. He said that painting was the one thing that made life worth living. He said that painting pain was a way of touching and being touched by a world he couldn't feel.

Practice guided by Parse's theory focuses on the experience of health for persons and families. The practice complements other disciplines in that it is based on a distinct knowledge base. No other discipline specifies knowledge about unitary human beings who live health as a process of becoming in relationship with others. The themes of meaning, rhythmical patterning, and transcendence when united in Parse's theory create a new system for understanding and interpreting the human-health interrelationship. Consider the following practice situation with a woman who attended a community center.

Parse's Theory with Person in Community Center

Janice visited the community center every day to eat and warm up a bit before heading back onto the street. She was a quiet woman and usually kept to herself. One day she started crying and while clutching a picture she looked at the nurse and said she did not know how she could make it through the day. The nurse asked Janice what was happening. Janice said her four-year-old child was very sick, that she might die. Rocking back and forth she said the pain of being without her child was unbearable. She explained that her child was in the care of foster parents and she wondered what she would do if her baby died before she got to see her again. The nurse was silently present as Janice paused before going on.

Janice said she was hurting, like a knife was in her heart. She spoke about a man who left her, an eviction notice, and the humiliation and shame of living in shelters and public houses. Janice was living in a boarding home where others had tuberculosis. A referral was made by someone, she does not know who, to social services and Janice was visited by a case worker who wanted to know about her child Sherry. The case worker talked to Janice about her inability to care for her child and Sherry was placed with foster parents. Janice said she could not fight for Sherry, that she wanted to do what was best and she felt so guilty for the way they had to live. She said she just had to let Sherry go and that the pain was going to rip her apart.

The nurse stayed with Janice without offering reassurances or suggestions. The nurse asked her to talk more about the pain. Janice said it was like having nails pounded into her. It was sharp and unending, it went everywhere and pain seeped out from her. Janice cried as she talked about the pain of being away from her child. After a few minutes she said, sometimes I wonder why I go on. The nurse asked Janice what kept her going on. Janice sat silently looking straight ahead for several minutes without saying a word and then she said, "I know I have some things I have to do. I have to get Sherry back with me and find some way to care for us." The nurse asked what she thought might help and Janice said she could not think of anything. Again the nurse was silently present. Suddenly Janice said she had one last option and that was to call her mother who lived 2000 miles away to see if she would let them both come home. Janice said this was really hard because she had not left her home on good terms and it had been ten years since she had visited her mother. Her mother did not even know Sherry, her only granddaughter. The nurse asked Janice if she could picture herself talking to her mother and what she might say to her. Janice began to shake as she said amidst sobs that she just wanted to ask if she could come home. At this point Janice left the center after thanking the nurse.

Janice returned to the center to talk to the nurse every week after this initial discussion. Sherry recovered from her illness and she continued to live with her foster parents. Janice talked to her case worker about making arrangements to call her mother and they were working toward some way to get herself and Sherry to her mother's home. Janice smiled when she left the center for the last time and she told the nurse she would not have been able to work things out if it had not been for the nurse's help. The help was the true presence lived by the nurse and experienced by the person; a presence that went with Janice's pain and anguish as well as her plans and hopes as she found her own way.

Parse's theory focuses on the person's/family's quality of life as it is defined and experienced by human beings themselves, and Parse's view of health is not defined according to medical illnesses, functional disabilities, or other standardized norms. The traditional biomedical theories define health first and then guide nurses to judge whether persons have it. The Parse nurse focuses in practice on the meaning of situations as described by persons in the context of their own unique lives. The way persons experience and participate in life situations and the daily happenings they contend with throughout life is of interest to the Parse nurse.

Health is a process, a continuous flow of ups and downs, losses and gains, joys and sorrows, successes and failures that relate to daily living. The nurse guided by Parse's theory participates in this process of living health. The changes that happen for persons who are with nurses guided by Parse's theory include: the illumination of meaning, the discovery of insights about self and others, the clarification of anticipated consequences, new understanding, and the identification of hopes and dreams. Persons in practice report enhanced quality of life related to the nurse's presence.

Parse identified a phenomenon she calls lingering presence that has also been reported in practice. It has been stated earlier that as nurses live true presence others illuminate meaning, synchronize rhythms, and move beyond. It is important to note that what is said and how meaning is described by persons is not for the benefit of the nurse. The nurse does not live true presence in order to collect information for various reasons. The nurse lives true presence because he or she knows that persons themselves will change the meaning and discover new things for themselves. The experience of being with a nurse who is truly present can surface a lingering presence that continues to be with the person through time, and that has important consequences. For example, a man said to a nurse he had not seen for two days: "I've been thinking a lot about what we talked about the other day and I've decided to go ahead and quit my job. You helped me to sort it out and I couldn't stop thinking about it." The nurse's presence made a difference in how the person worked through the complexities of a difficult job situation.

CONCLUSION

Parse's theory of human becoming presents an opportunity for nurses to learn and commit to a different way of nursing. It is a theory that focuses on the inherent value of human beings and their unique unfolding or human becoming, which is health. The practice of Parse's theory is learned over time in the living of true presence. The goal of practice is quality of life as defined by persons themselves.

The mark of a growing discipline is the emergence of different ways of thinking and acting in relation to a central phenomenon of concern. Nursing is pushing its boundaries and extending its roots to grow beyond. The study of universal experiences guided by Parse's theory will enhance understanding and expand the knowledge base for practice. Nurses endorsing the traditional empirical paradigm and its related causal approaches argue that understanding does not translate into do-able interventions. This is true. A scientific base, like that housed in Parse's theory, that enhances understanding will only change horizons, broaden perspectives, and expand respect for human diversity. These changes do not relate to what nurses do to people but to how nurses think about human beings and their unfolding health. Understanding changes patterns of relating and it is precisely patterns of relating in the nurse-person relationship that influence quality of life. Parse's theory is a symbol of growth, a sign of change that contributes to nursing science in a unique and influential way.

REFERENCES

Banonis, B. C. (1989). The lived experience of recovering from addiction: A phenomenological study. *Nursing Science Quarterly, 2,* 37–43.

Butler, M. J. (1988). Family transformation: Parse's theory in practice. *Nursing Science Quarterly, 1,* 68–74.

Butler, M. J., & Snodgrass, F. G. (1991). Beyond abuse: Parse's theory in practice. *Nursing Science Quarterly, 4,* 76–82.

Cody, W. K. (1991). Grieving a personal loss. *Nursing Science Quarterly, 4,* 61–68.

Cody, W. K. (1992). *The meaning of grieving for families living with AIDS.* Unpublished doctoral dissertation. University of South Carolina, Columbia, SC.

Cody, W. K., & Mitchell, G. J. (1992). Parse's theory of nursing: The cutting edge. *Advances in Nursing Science, 15*(2), 52–65.

Cowling, W. R. (1989). Parse's theory of nursing. In J. J. Fitzpatrick & A. L. Whall (Eds.), *Conceptual models on nursing: Analysis and application* (pp. 385–399). (2nd ed.). Bowie, MD: Brady.

Dilthey, W. (1976). *Selected writings* (H. P. Rickman, Ed. and Trans.). New York: Harper & Row.

Dilthey, W. (1977). The understanding of other persons and their expressions of life. (Original work published 1927). In R. M. Zaner &

K. L. Heiges (Trans.), *Descriptive psychology and historical understanding* (pp. 123–144). The Hague, Netherlands: Nijhoff.

Ermarth, M. (1978). *Wilhelm Dilthey: The critique of historical reason.* Chicago: University of Chicago Press.

Giorgi, A. (1970). *Psychology as a human science.* New York: Harper & Row.

Giorgi, A. (1985). Sketch of a psychological phenomenological method. In A. Giorgi (Ed.), *Phenomenology and psychological research* (pp. 8–22). Pittsburgh: Duquesne University Press.

Grudin, R. (1990). *The grace of great things—creativity and innovation.* New York: Ticknor & Fields.

Heidegger, M. (1962). *Being and time* (J. Macquarrie & E. Robinson, Trans.). New York: Harper & Row.

Jonas, C. M. (1992). The lived experience of being an elder in Nepal. *Nursing Science Quarterly, 5,* 171–176.

Jourard, S. (1972). Some notes on the experience of commitment. *Humanitas, VIII*(1), 5–8.

Kelley, L. M. (1991). Struggling with going along when you do not believe. *Nursing Science Quarterly, 4,* 123–129.

Kockelmans, J. J. (1985). *Heidegger and science.* Washington, DC: Center for Advanced Research in Phenomenology & University Press of America.

Mattice, M. (1991). Parse's theory of nursing in practice: A manager's perspective. *Canadian Journal of Nursing Administration, 4*(1), 11–13.

Mattice, M., & Mitchell, G. J. (1990). Caring for confused elders: Evaluating our methods of orientation. *The Canadian Nurse, 86*(11), 16–18.

Mitchell, G. J. (1986). Utilizing Parse's theory of man-living-health in Mrs. M's neighborhood. *Perspectives, 10*(4), 5–7.

Mitchell, G. J. (1988). Man-living-health: The theory in practice. *Nursing Science Quarterly, 1,* 120–127.

Mitchell, G. J. (1990a). The lived experience of taking life day-by-day in later life: Research guided by Parse's emergent method. *Nursing Science Quarterly*, *3*, 29–36.

Mitchell, G. J. (1990b). Struggling in change: From the traditional approach to Parse's theory-based practice. *Nursing Science Quarterly*, *3*, 170–176.

Mitchell, G. J. (1991). Nursing diagnosis: An ethical analysis. *IMAGE: Journal of Nursing Scholarship*, *23*(2), 99–103.

Mitchell, G. J. (1992). *Exploring the paradoxical experience of restriction-freedom in later life: Parse's theory-guided research.* Unpublished doctoral dissertation. University of South Carolina, Columbia, SC.

Mitchell, G. J., & Cody, W. K. (1992). Nursing knowledge and human science: Ontological and epistemological considerations. *Nursing Science Quarterly*, *5*, 54–61.

Mitchell, G. J., & Copplestone, C. (1990). Applying Parse's theory to perioperative nursing: A nontraditional approach. *AORN Journal*, *51*(3), 787–798.

Mitchell G. J., & Pilkington, B. (1990). Theoretical approaches in nursing: A comparison of Roy and Parse. *Nursing Science Quarterly*, *3*, 81–87.

Mitchell, G. J., & Santopinto, M. D. A. (1988). An alternative to nursing diagnosis. *The Canadian Nurse*, *84*(10), 25–28.

Nagle, L., & Mitchell, G. J. (1991). Theoretic diversity: Evolving paradigmatic issues in research and practice. *Advances in Nursing Science*, *14*(1), 17–25.

Nokes, N. K., & Carver, K. (1991). The meaning of living with AIDS: A study using Parse's theory of man-living-health. *Nursing Science Quarterly*, *4*, 174–179.

Parse, R. R. (1981). *Man-living-health: A theory of nursing.* New York: Wiley.

Parse, R. R. (1987). *Nursing science: Major paradigms, theories, and critiques.* Philadelphia: Saunders.

Parse, R. R. (1990a). Health: A personal commitment. *Nursing Science Quarterly*, *3*, 136–140.

Parse, R. R. (1990b). Parse's research methodology with an illustration of the lived experience of hope. *Nursing Science Quarterly, 3*, 9–17.

Parse, R. R. (1992a). Human becoming: Parse's theory of nursing. *Nursing Science Quarterly, 5*, 35–42.

Parse, R. R. (1992b). *Research and practice methodologies of Parse's theory.* Paper presented at the second annual Parse's conference. Killington, Vermont. October 23–25.

Parse, R. R., Coyne, A. B., & Smith, M. J. (1985). *Nursing research: Qualitative methods.* Bowie, MD: Brady.

Phillips, J. R. (1987). A critique of Parse's man-living-health theory. In R. R. Parse (Ed.), *Nursing science: Major paradigms, theories, and critiques* (pp. 181–204). Philadelphia: Saunders.

Pilkington, F. B. (In Press). The lived experience of grieving the loss of an important other. *Nursing Science Quarterly.*

Polkinghorne, D. E. (1983). Methodology for the human sciences. Albany, NY: State University of New York Press.

Quiquero, A., Knights, D., & Meo, O. (1991). Theory as a guide to practice: Staff nurses choose Parse's theory. *Canadian Journal of Nursing Administration, 4*(1), 14–16.

Rasmusson, D. L., Jonas, C. M., & Mitchell, G. J. (1991). The eye of the beholder: Parse's theory with homeless individuals. *Clinical Nurse Specialist, 5*, 139–143.

Santopinto, M. D. A. (1989). The relentless drive to be ever thinner: A study using the phenomenological method. *Nursing Science Quarterly, 2*, 29–36.

Smith, M. C. (1990). Struggling through a difficult time for unemployed persons. *Nursing Science Quarterly, 3*, 18–28.

Smith, M. C. (1991). Existential–phenomenological foundations in nursing: A discussion of differences. *Nursing Science Quarterly, 4*, 5–6.

Smith, M. C., & Heudopohl, J. H. (1990). Analysis and evaluation of Parse's theory of man-living-health. *Canadian Journal of Nursing Research, 20*(4), 43–57.

Wondolowski, C., & Davis, D. K. (1988). The lived experience of aging in the oldest old: A phenomenological study. *The American Journal of Psychoanalysis, 48,* 261–270.

Wondolowski, C., & Davis, D. K. (1991). The lived experience of health in the oldest old: A phenomenological study. *Nursing Science Quarterly, 4,* 113–118.

Part IV

Nursing as Caring Theory

7

Nursing as Caring: An Emerging General Theory of Nursing

Savina O. Schoenhofer
Anne Boykin

The purpose of this chapter is to explore how the theory of Nursing as Caring influences nursing practice. A full understanding of the implications presented requires an in-depth understanding of the theory and its underlying assumptions. Presentation of the full theory is beyond the scope of this chapter. The theory, Nursing as Caring, should be studied in its entirety for the fullness of meaning (Boykin & Schoenhofer, 1993). Only major ideas from the theory will be presented, followed by questions frequently asked by nurses in practice.

The unique focus of nursing is posited as "nurturing persons living caring and growing in caring." This perspective of the focus of nursing comes from a fundamental view of caring as the human mode of being (Roach, 1984, 1987). Nursing as Caring builds on this foundation by recognizing personhood as a process of living grounded in caring and that personhood is enhanced through participation in nurturing relationships with caring others. Persons are viewed as already complete and continuously growing in completeness, fully caring and unfolding caring possibilities moment-to-moment. Being complete in the moment means that there is no insufficiency, no brokenness nor absence of something. Nursing activities are not directed toward "healing" in the sense of making whole; from our perspective, wholeness is present and unfolding. There is no lack, failure, or inadequacy which is to be corrected through nursing.

The concept of nursing situation is central to every aspect of

Nursing as Caring. We have claimed that all nursing knowledge re-
sides within the nursing situation (Boykin & Schoenhofer, 1991). The
nursing situation is known as a lived experience in which the caring
between the nurse and the one nursed celebrates and enhances personhood. The nurse brings to the nursing situation self as caring person. It
is within the nursing situation that the nurse comes to know the other
as caring person, living unique ways of caring and growing in caring.
When a situation is approached from the perspective of Nursing as Caring, person is understood to be a caring person, living caring in his or
her everyday life. The nurse enters into the world of the other person
with the intention of knowing the other as caring person. It is in knowing the other in their "living caring and growing in caring" that calls for
nursing are heard. A call for nursing is a call for specific forms of caring
which acknowledge, affirm, and sustain the other as they strive to live
caring uniquely. Knowing the other in this way means coming to know
how the other is living caring in the situation and expressing aspirations
for growing in caring. The call for nursing is a call for specific caring
responses which will sustain and enhance the other's unique process of
living caring and growing in caring in the situation. This is the caring
nurturance which we call the nursing response. The caring response
called forth in each nursing situation is created for that moment.

Nursing as Caring is a theory of nursing born in practice and intended as a framework for practice in the real world of nursing. Professional practice is a special and particular social commitment that goes
beyond everyday social interaction. When a person in the role of nurse
offers nursing service to another, that offer is an offer to care. The
practice of Nursing as Caring calls for the nurse to relinquish adherence
to concepts which bind and limit nursing to health-illness (or wellness-
illness) frameworks. For the nurse practicing Nursing as Caring, it is
necessary to form an intent to develop and maintain a perspective of
coming to know persons as caring. That is, an understanding of the
focus of nursing as nurturing persons living caring and growing in caring
is the basis for practicing from this framework.

QUESTIONS NURSES ASK ABOUT NURSING AS CARING

How does the nurse come to know self and other as caring person?
The person of nurse has been in the process of knowing self as

caring person since the earliest moment of knowing. The process of enhancing competence in living caring occurs over a lifetime, and can occur in very subtle ways. Inherent in the preceding question is the notion of deliberately knowing self and other as caring. Styles (1982) in her book, *On Nursing: Toward a New Endowment*, stresses the relationship of professionhood to the profession. Professionhood is described as comprising the characteristics of the individual who is a member of the profession. The profession is the collective consciousness of nursing, while professionhood is the way in which a nurse lives out nursing day to day. It is important to reflect on who we are as persons for it is the person who assumes the multifaceted roles of nurse.

How does one come to know self as caring person? Mayeroff's (1971) caring ingredients are useful conceptual tools when the nurse is struggling to know self and other as caring. Ingredients such as honesty, courage, hope, and knowing may be discovered in the moment as the nurse offers to care. Other caring ingredients which might serve as a bridge between two persons include trust, honesty, humility, and alternating rhythm.

All relationships are opportunities to draw forth caring possibilities, opportunities to reinforce the beauty of person-as-person. Through honestly knowing self, I am able to be authentic to self and others. I am able to see from the inside what others see from the outside. Whatever feelings, attitudes, and actions are lived in the moment, they are matched by an inner genuine awareness. The more I am open to knowing and appreciating self and trying to understand the world of the other, the greater the awareness of our interconnectedness as caring persons. One may come to better know self as caring person by:

- Trusting in self; freeing self up to become what one can truly become, and valuing self.

- Learning to let go, to transcend—to let go of problems, difficulties, in order to remember the interconnectedness that enables us to know self and other as living caring, even in suffering and in seeking relief from suffering.

- Being open and humble enough to experience and know self to be at home with one's feelings.

- Continuously calling to consciousness that each person is living caring in the moment and we are each developing uniquely in our becoming.

- Taking time to fully experience our humanness for one can only truly understand in another what one can understand in self.

- Finding hope in the moment.

Must I like my patients to nurse them?

It is useful to consider the related question: What does it mean to dislike someone? Does it mean that one is unable to know the other as caring? Is it possible to dislike some or even most of the life choices another makes, and still care for the person? The commitment to know another as caring person in order to nurse him or her is the challenge which makes nursing special among all professions. So the answer to the question about liking my patient is yes. As nurse I must find some basis for connecting with the other as caring person. Without connecting or without entering the world of the other in order to know the other as caring person, there can be no mutual process engendering respect. The result of not taking the risk to know other is objectification of other. What comes across is non-nursing, that is, dislike, judgmental disapproval, coldness, or insincerity.

Why is it essential that I find a basis of connecting with other as caring person? Because to understand another's call for caring is to understand how the other is living caring in the moment and living hopes and dreams for growing in caring. It is in this understanding that the nurse creates caring uniquely in the moment. It is this unique creating of caring in the person-to-person situation that is the nursing response.

Is it possible to nurse one who is in an unconscious state of awareness?

We have asserted that all nursing takes place in nursing situations. A nursing situation is a shared lived experience in which the caring between nurse and the one nursed enhances personhood. It may be asked, can a nursing situation exist when the one nursed is unconscious. It may be difficult to understand how the nurse could enter the world of the unconscious person, how there could be *caring between* the nurse and the one nursed in this situation.

When nursing a person who is unconscious, the nurse lives the commitment to know the other as caring person. How is that commitment lived? It requires that all ways of knowing be brought into action. The nurse must make self as caring person available to the one nursed. The fullness of the nurse as caring person is called forth. This requires use of Mayeroff's caring ingredients: the alternating rhythm of knowing about the other and knowing the other directly through authentic presence and attunement; the hope and courage to risk opening self to one who cannot communicate verbally, patiently trusting in self to understand the other's mode of living caring in the moment; honest humility as one brings all that one knows and remains open to learning from the other. The nurse attuned to the other as person might for example experience the vulnerability of the person who lies unconscious from surgical anesthetic or traumatic injury. In that vulnerability, the nurse recognizes that the one nursed is living caring in humility, hope and trust. Instead of responding to the vulnerability, merely "taking care of" the other, the nurse practicing Nursing as Caring might respond by honoring the other's humility, by participating in the other's hopefulness, by steadfast trustworthiness. Creating caring in the moment in this situation might come from the nurse resonating with past and present personal experiences of vulnerability. Connected to this form of personal knowing might be an ethical knowing that power as a reciprocal of vulnerability can develop undesirable status differential in the nurse-patient role relationship. As the nurse sifts through a myriad of empirical data, the most significant information emerges—this is a *person* with whom I am called to care. Ethical knowing again merges with other pathways as the nurse forms the decision to go beyond vulnerability and engage the other as caring person, not helpless object of another's concern. Aesthetic knowing comes in the praxis of caring, in living chosen ways of honoring humility, joining in hope, and demonstrating trustworthiness in the moment.

What about nursing a person for whom it is difficult to care?

Sometimes what nurses *do* is taken out of the context of what nursing *is*. When that happens, it seems that nurses offer to perform tasks related to medically prescribed treatments or carry out norm-based illness-preventing activities. Caring in nursing is viewed as a mutual human process in which the nurse artistically responds with authentic presence to a call for nursing (Boykin & Schoenhofer, 1990). Treatments are carried out, tasks performed, but no nursing has been given without a specific intent to care. Genuine nursing requires more than this. As we understand it, nursing *is* caring, and without caring, no nursing occurs.

When the nurse practices from the perspective of nursing as nurturing persons living caring and growing in caring, the nurse enters the situation committed to caring. This means that the nurse engages the other with the purpose of knowing the other as caring person.

Potential nursing situations where the one to be nursed has committed an act which is universally condemned as inhuman, present a conceptual and practical problem. We see this problem as a challenge, a challenge to the nurse's commitment to care. For example, in nursing a parent who has abused a child, or a person who has sexually molested a child, or a person who has committed multiple gruesome murders, the nurse's commitment to care is strongly challenged by the horror of the acts committed by the one to be nursed. What is called for in such situations is not that the nurse ignore nor approve the inhuman act, but that the nurse seek to know the other as caring person. This requires transcending the knowing which is pre-existing, the knowing about other as noncaring. Transcending differs from setting aside or bracketing the immediate. If one were to set aside knowledge of the inhuman act, for example, knowledge that this person I am to nurse has tortured his infant child, caring would not be genuine. I as nurse practicing Nursing as Caring would be called upon to live my commitment to knowing the other as caring, and that means knowing the other in the moment. For me to know the other in the moment, it is necessary to look beyond the past into the present and keep the moment alive with human possibility. What else is there to do? One cannot *nurse* from anger, horror, or from despising another. To nurse, one must recognize the humanness in the face of inhumanness. That is what it means to transcend.

Extreme cases of child molestation, torture, and genocide differ only in degree from the usual nursing situations which present themselves. In nursing another, there is always the potential for the nurse to discover some undesirable characteristic or a fundamental value difference. The degree of challenge presented from situation to situation may vary but the commitment is steadfast, to know the other as caring person. How the nurse manages to live this commitment is to know self as caring person, to have the willingness and ability to transcend one's own limitations, even inhumanity, to find the humanity and caring in oneself, and to hold this commitment as worthwhile.

It often takes courage for those known to have committed a seriously antisocial act to present themselves for care. It is frequently an expression of hope as well. Courage and hope, when recognized by the nurse, activate a connection between two caring persons. When this connection is realized in the mind of the nurse, nursing has begun.

Practicing Nursing as Caring does not require that the nurse be super-human. It does require, however, that the nurse have a depth and breadth of knowledge of caring. This knowledge must be alive and growing through the use of multiple pathways of knowing. If caring is the nurse's expertise (Boykin & Schoenhofer, 1991), it follows that the nurse must not only be schooled in caring, but must also be involved in an ongoing process of growing in awareness of self as caring person. Difficult nursing situations like those posed above are opportunities for the nurse to expand a personal sense of self as caring person and a repertoire of caring expressions.

How does the nursing process fit with this theory?

Many nursing theories developed in the past two decades were grounded in the linear problem-solving process which Orlando (1961) termed the nursing process. An assumption of the nursing process is that one will be making decisions for others, or at least making decisions as a basis for taking action on behalf of others. Another assumption of nursing process is that decision making is preferable to choice, and is based primarily on rational analysis of empirical data. A further assumption is that other ways of knowing are unverifiable and therefore invalid. In fact, the nursing process was an effort to develop nursing as a science, partly in reaction to an over-reliance on nursing as an art. The limits of utility of logical empiricism are becoming apparent. There is a move in nursing to re-own the art, to transcend the artificial polarization of art vs. science, and to discover the profound unity that is nursing.

The process of coming to know other and the process of nursing cannot be expressed in the traditional linear nursing process format. Generally what is reflected in the nursing process is information which is rooted in the disciplines of biology, chemistry, medicine, psychology and sociology. In the nursing process format, the guide for nursing is largely textbook knowledge rather than knowledge gleaned from knowing the person as person.

From the perspective of Nursing as Caring, the nurse enters a nursing situation with the purpose of knowing other as caring person. Because the person is viewed as complete, the nurse would not attempt to know other through a fragmented, system-type approach. The process of nursing is focused on nurturing persons living caring and growing in caring. Through entering the world of the nursed, the nurse comes to know the calls for nursing. The nurse would not attempt to use a 'label' or a diagnosis to describe the situation of nursing. There are no labels that could do this. The reason for nursing could be described only in terms of the unique calls for nursing which are being heard in the situation. The calls for nursing would be shared with colleagues and each nurse would respond to the calls in ways which uniquely reflect who the nurse is as caring person.

Much of what happens in nursing situations is neither measurable nor empirically verifiable. That which is measurable and empirically verifiable is relevant in the situation, however, and may be called upon at any time to contribute to and through the nurse's empirical knowing. Information which the nurse has available becomes knowledge within the nursing situation. Knowing the person directly is what guides the selection and patterning of relevant points of factual information in a nursing situation. That is, any fact or set of facts from nursing research or related bodies of information can be considered for relevance and drawn into the supporting knowledge base. This knowledge base remains open and evolving as the nurse employs an alternating rhythm of scanning and considering facts for relevance while remaining grounded in the nursing situation.

What are the assumptions on which this theory is based?

To understand the practical implications of Nursing as Caring, it is necessary to understand the assumptions on which the theory is built. Some important assumptions include:

- caring is the human mode of being (Roach, 1984; 1987);
- caring is lived by each person, moment to moment;
- personhood is a process of living grounded in caring;
- personhood is enhanced through participating in nurturing relationships with caring others;
- nursing is for celebrating and enhancing personhood, not for correcting failures or deficiencies.

Thus, the nurse operates from a fundamental assumption that, while persons express many characteristics, caring is the most human of them.

Further, this assumption means that while other ways of being may be lived, the essence of what it means to be human is somehow simultaneously present. While recognizing the other as caring person is sometimes a difficult challenge, it is the commitment which guides the practicing nurse. The nurse approaches the other with the intent to come to know the other as living caring in the moment and expressing hopes and dreams for growing in caring.

Together with this commitment and intent, the nurse must undertake a lifelong study of caring. While caring is the human mode of being, abilities to recognize and express caring can be developed. The study of caring is enhanced when one opens multiple pathways of knowing. Personal knowing of caring is that knowing which comes from experiences of being cared for and an awareness of one's own expressions of caring in a wide range of relationships and situations. Knowledge of caring can expand through contact with the growing literature on caring in nursing and related fields (Boykin & Schoenhofer, 1990; Morse, Solberg, Neander, Bottorff, & Johnson, 1990; Smerke, 1989). Weighing the various meanings of caring in situations and making choices for expressing caring, contributes too, to deepening understanding. Aesthetic knowing of caring, creating and appreciating the meaning of caring in embodied situations is perhaps the pathway to fully knowing caring, to fully knowing self and other as caring persons.

The value of the theory, Nursing as Caring, is that it is born in nursing. It provides a framework for viewing nursing practice which embodies the values of appreciating person-as-person and knowing the fullness of other as caring person. The focus of nursing is clearly articulated. Each of these points of value are illustrated in the following chapter which presents the application of the theory Nursing as Caring.

REFERENCES

Boykin, A., & Schoenhofer, S. (1993). *Nursing as caring: A model for revolutionizing practice.* New York: National League for Nursing Press.

Boykin, A., & Schoenhofer, S. (1991). Story as link between nursing practice, ontology, epistemology. *Image, 23,* 245–248.

Boykin, A., & Schoenhofer, S. (1990). Caring in nursing: Analysis of extant theory. *Nursing Science Quarterly, 4,* 149–155.

Mayeroff, M. (1971). *On caring*. New York: Harper & Row.

Morse, J., Solberg, S., Neander, W., Bottorff, J., & Johnson, J. (1990). Concepts of caring and caring as a concept. *Advances in Nursing Science*, *13*(1), 1–14.

Orlando, I. (1961). *The dynamic nurse-patient-relationship: Function, process, and principles*. New York: G.P. Putnam's Sons.

Roach, S. (1984). *Caring: The human mode of being, implications for nursing*. Toronto: Faculty of Nursing, University of Toronto. (Perspectives in Caring Monograph 1).

Roach, S. (1987). *The human act of caring*. Ottawa: Canadian Hospital Association.

Smerke, J. (1989). *Interdisciplinary guide to the literature for human caring*. New York: National League for Nursing Press. Publication No. 15-2331.

Styles, M. (1982). *On nursing: Toward a new endowment*. St. Louis: Mosby.

8

Practical Applications of Nursing
As Caring Theory

Carol Kearney
Vicki Yeager

The personal interpretations of the Nursing As Caring theory in this chapter represent our search for balance and harmony in our respective nursing practices. For us, this has been an evolutionary process of affirming and reaffirming self and other. The Nursing As Caring theory has guided us to the ultimate freedom of taking responsibility for the knowing of self and other.

It is within the nursing situation that the nurse comes to know other. The nursing situation is known as a shared, lived experience in which the caring between the nurse and the one nursed celebrates and enhances personhood (Boykin & Schoenhofer, 1993). The nurse joins in the life process of the person nursed, and brings his or her life process to the relationship as well.

In this chapter we share personal stories that describe nursing situations we have lived in our individual nursing practices. These particular stories were chosen because of the richness of how they illustrate the theory, Nursing As Caring. Following the stories, we present four major themes of the theory and share our thoughts about how these themes have guided us in our practice of Nursing As Caring.

NURSING STORIES

Carol's Story:
It was 3:00 P.M. I closed the curtain and helped Mrs. Clarke to the chair for her bath. She was a 68-year-old grandmother who had been

93

admitted the day before with a bleeding gastric ulcer and hemoglobin of 4.2. When I first met her in the early morning, she complained of a headache and I found her blood pressure to be dangerously high. She asked me to let her sleep, which she did most of the morning after I medicated her. In the early afternoon I spent time with her and her husband answering questions about and explaining the need for her I.V., medications, and clear liquid diet. She was very relieved when I told her she could walk in the hall with the I.V. pole.

As I placed a basin filled with warm water on her table and helped take off her nightgown I sensed her tension. Her gown was from home. It was soft like silk, with lace along the neckline. The telemetry wires poking out from her chest seemed out of place. As I put the I.V. bag through the arm of her gown I said, "I'll help you with your back if you'd like." She said, "Thank you. That would be nice." As I began washing her back, I smelled lilac perfume and then a faint scent of cigarette smoke. I thought for a moment, and decided I needed to ask her about the smoke. "I love that lilac perfume you have on, Mrs. Clarke," I commented. She responded, "Oh, you smell that? I don't smell it." I followed with, "I also smell cigarette smoke. Have you been smoking?" She immediately turned to me, and in a desperate voice said, "Yes, but please don't tell anyone, please." Having no time to think about my response, I put my hand on her shoulder and said, "I won't tell anyone, but I am concerned. Does your doctor know you're smoking in the hospital?" "No, and don't tell him, he'd be furious!" she answered emphatically.

As I dried her back, I repeated, "I promise I won't tell anyone about your smoking, it's between you and me. But I do feel that I have a responsibility to tell you that you're taking a risk smoking, especially when your blood pressure is elevated, as it was this morning. If you have to smoke, you need to be very careful. It isn't safe smoking in your room, because of the oxygen. There are no designated smoking areas in this hospital." She quickly responded, "I've been going down to the visitors bathroom – they smoke in there, too."

I now understood why she had been so relieved in the morning when I told her she could walk in the hall with her I.V. pole. As I rubbed lotion on her back, there were a few moments of silence. Mrs. Clarke then asked, "Is there anywhere I can go? I have to smoke—I only take a few puffs, it's the only way I can relax! I really want to go home." I told her again there were no designated smoking areas, but if she chose to smoke, the visitors bathroom was probably the best place. She took the wash cloth and began washing her face. I told her, "I'll let you finish your bath and I'll be back in a few minutes to help you with your clean gown." As I stepped toward the door she again said, "Please don't tell anyone." I looked right at her and said, "Mrs. Clarke, I will not tell anyone. Just be careful." "Thank you," she answered.

As I was leaving the room, I realized that I had made a decision against hospital policy and a decision that could be dangerous to her health. But I knew I had made the right decision. During the last few hours of my shift, I saw her walking in the hallway several times. She did not speak about her smoking again, but later was very anxious to show me pictures of her new granddaughter. I visited Mrs. Clarke one more time and told her that I would be going home soon, and that a new nurse would be with her for the night. As I was completing the flow sheet at the end of her bed, she said, "Thank you for being so kind. Thank you for everything." I knew what she meant by 'everything.' I thought about our situation together, again, during report at the end of the shift. Ten years ago, right out of nursing school, I would have been very uncomfortable not telling the nurse or doctor about her smoking. But rather than revealing our secret to her oncoming nurse, I kept it hidden in my heart.

This particular nursing situation demonstrates how the theory of Nursing As Caring can be applied in everyday nursing practice. Although unique, it was not one of those situations that occurs once in a lifetime. Rather, this was the kind of situation that all nurses have experienced with their patients in a variety of health care settings. It is often during those shared moments when the nurse is helping a patient with a simple task, such as bathing, or doing a nursing procedure that the nurse is able to 'enter the world of the other.' My short time with Mrs. Clarke allowed me to know her as a caring person and to understand what was important to her.

Vicki's Story:

The phone call came on Sunday morning. "Won't you please take on a private case that begins tomorrow?" "Is the patient dying?" I ask. "Oh, no, only an elderly lady who has had a recent colostomy. She just needs a nurse for a few days so she can adjust to the colostomy before she goes home." Accepting the assignment, I know the true meaning of this call is not about colostomies. It is about the dance of life which has as its rhythm, the elemental human need of caring about and caring for another. Yes, learning about colostomies will happen, evolving from the knowing of the other.

Monday morning, the hospital is quiet. The staff nurse meets me outside your room and is obviously relieved that you have a private duty nurse. She tells me that you're rather demanding and difficult. The rest of report is a recitation of I.V. infusion rates, Morphine Sulfate dosages, I & O's, etc. As I listen to report I'm trying to keep you focused as a whole, rather than all the parts just now thrown at me. Walking into your darkened room, I am surprised by your size. Small and asleep in the hospital bed, your open mouth breaths drag in great gulps of life. You, "the difficult one," have fists clenched at your sides. Will you be telling me about this anger? There, you stir, and as a fist unclenches, I slip my hand in yours. Do your pale bony fingers feel the rapid pulse of my heart? Your eyes start open, releasing a frown. "Hello," you say, "you must be the nurse, I'm Lois." The connection was made, and so began our awesome knowing.

The next two weeks we spent learning this dance of life. Most times you would lead, occasionally we would both try to lead and always you sang your song of going home. When we had figured out some basic dance steps, you told me about your anger. And it was about dying. So when the hospice nurse came to talk about the inevitable hospice home visits, you and I became serious about our dance music. Raising the volume of our silent music we were able to drown out her painful words disguised as comforting Muzak, words like "palliative support measures." Dying and death were left unspoken.

After the nurse had left, you looked at me straight on and told me you hadn't understood a single word she had said. "But, will you go home with me?", you asked. In the space of a few seconds you had disavowed and affirmed your knowing. And of course I agreed to go home with you.

Home. Normalcy. Stability. Lifetime habits resumed. Morning crossword puzzles, the ritual of lipstick, one martini lunches, writing letters and always giving specific instructions about everything. Meantime, we just kept upping your narcotic dosage to keep the pain at bay. Because, who knows, maybe the center will hold. I know that is what I wanted to believe.

But then one afternoon before your nap, you asked me if you were ever going to get any better. And I had to tell you, "No, I don't think you will." I sat on your bed and held your hand as I said those words. You looked back at me with your level gaze and said, "Well, I'm glad you told me." Had you seen the sadness in my eyes? Did I give myself away so easily to you?

At the end you were so tired. There were moments when anything seemed possible. But only moments. We talked about me leaving for my long planned holiday. You told me you wished I wasn't going, but knew I must. And I really didn't want to leave you. I told you so. That last day I whispered to you that I wanted to take you with me. We hugged. You, austere and loving, telling me you so looked forward to my return. Walking out of your house, I looked back. Your level gaze looked me straight on as my throat closed around the last good-bye.

The Nursing As Caring theory has at its core a deliberate acknowledgment of the completeness of self and other (Boykin & Schoenhofer, 1993). Within this situation there is no 'diagnosis' on which to focus. There is no wrong to right. Rather, the Nursing As Caring theory acknowledges and celebrates completeness by recognizing all human emotion and interaction as essential components of the lived experience between the participants. Consequently, Lois' story is an affirmation of the completeness of person, a completeness that includes pain, laughter, hope, anger, trust, honesty, and death. All enhance the lived experience. Through the telling and retelling of the story, Lois continues to live and grow with me. My growth in personhood is enhanced as I continue to examine the meaning of my life within this unique nursing situation.

THEMES OF NURSING AS CARING

We have identified four major themes within the Nursing As Caring theory which guide us in our practice of the theory. Each theme will be presented in the form of a question and followed by our unique responses to these questions, thus guiding the reader's understanding of the theory in practice.

In our unique nursing situations, how did we see the other as caring person?

Carol: I believe one of the most difficult aspects of this nursing theory is knowing the other as caring person. Caring for patients who are hostile, have done something we think is wrong, or who cannot communicate with us is very challenging. Knowing how they are living caring in any particular moment can be even more difficult.

All human beings are caring (Boykin & Schoenhofer, 1993). Therefore, I knew Mrs. Clarke was caring and it was my intention to determine how she was living caring with me. I believe she was living caring in several unique ways. In his book, On Caring, Mayeroff (1971) says that to be a caring person means living the meaning of one's own life. This involves being open and living congruence between one's beliefs and behaviors. Mrs. Clarke believed smoking cigarettes was the only way she could relax in the hospital. She was acting on her belief, and therefore, was caring.

She was living caring through her openness and honesty with me. In revealing her smoking she showed a willingness to let me into her life at that moment, to see her struggle with being sick in the hospital, and to understand the importance of cigarettes to her. She showed courage and trust in our relationship. Although she was afraid that her doctor would learn of her secret and that she would not be able to smoke, she was courageous in her admission that she had been smoking. She believed that I would not tell her secret, and that I would accept her and her decision to smoke. Mrs. Clarke's openness and trust made it easier for me to see her as a caring person.

Vicki: I came to know Lois as a caring person over many days and weeks. Caring did not leap out and announce itself. It was present in many guises, sometimes palpable, soft, and relaxed, sometimes steely, controlled, and angry. It was always there, waiting to be distinguished as caring. I began to examine how Lois was living trust, honesty, humility and courage, and I found caring manifested therein.

When narcotic dosages were increased, Lois offered herself over to the amorphous haze of non-pain. How courageous of her, going into that unknown, and how humble of her to acknowledge that she could not bear the pain without the narcotics. She was caring through her honesty in trying to keep daily rituals intact, hope that the rituals would keep stability at the center of her life, and trust in asking me if she would ever get any better and that my answer and her response would be authentic. We passed through that incredible moment with the self-realization of living intensely in the moment.

How did we enter the world of other with the intention of knowing other?

Carol: The Nursing As Caring theory describes people, 'persons,' as being whole or complete, rather than being broken, or having problems and deficiencies (Boykin & Schoenhofer, 1993). This perspective suggests that the nurse's role is to support and nurture persons as they grow in completeness. Understanding my role from this perspective and appreciating the completeness of Mrs. Clarke helped me to enter into her world with the intention of knowing her as caring person. I did not view her as a weak, nervous lady with a smoking problem. Rather, I saw her as an open, honest, and courageous person calling for my acceptance and support of the way she chose to live her life. Knowing her as caring person clarified my understanding of her call and guided my nursing response with her.

Knowing myself as caring person also helped me to enter her world. Years of practical experience and a graduate education have given me more confidence to be open and honest with my patients. I have learned the importance of taking risks, of 'going out on a limb' for my patients. Most importantly, I have learned the uniqueness and beauty of each nursing situation and the power of my caring response. I felt comfortable asking Mrs. Clarke about her smoking, accepting her, and keeping our secret because that was my way of living caring with her.

Vicki: As I entered Lois' world, her courage, trust and hope as caring person were uniquely known. Her courageous questioning of me about her illness required that I too live courageously. My response that I didn't think she would get better took us into the unknown, enhancing our trust with one another. By participating in daily rituals with Lois, I helped her keep hope that her life continue to have purpose and that a sense of centeredness would prevail, as cancer spread inexorably from ovaries to colon to bone. She lived her life according to her beliefs that daily rituals were a necessity to her. I now understood why her one martini lunches, daily crossword puzzles, and frequent letter writing were of much importance to her.

What were the special calls for caring nurturance in our nursing situations?

Carol: In coming to know the other as caring person, the nurse hears calls for nursing, which originate within the unique relationship of the nursing situation. A call for nursing is a call for specific forms of caring, which acknowledge, affirm, and sustain the other as they strive to live caring uniquely (Boykin & Schoenhofer, 1993). I heard Mrs. Clarke's call for caring when she admitted her smoking to me. She was calling for knowledge and understanding of her situation and what smoking meant to her situation. Most importantly, her call was for my acceptance and nurturance of her as a person, and for my support of her decision to smoke.

Vicki: I conceptualized the call for caring nurturance as Lois' desire to live her life as a continuum and not as an end. Lois' disagreement with the hospice nurse's plan for her care ordered my caring response with her. I knew then that we would never discuss death and that her wish to stay at home with dignity was her way of living caring.

What were the unique forms of caring nurturance that enhanced personhood in these nursing situations?

Carol: The unique forms of caring nurturance expressed in the nursing situation are called the nursing responses (Boykin & Schoenhofer, 1993). These responses are the nurse's personal expressions of caring. Each nurse brings a unique perspective and understanding of self and of caring to each nursing situation, which affects the way the nurse responds to calls for caring nurturance. Vicki and I have had diverse educational and practical experiences. We perceive caring differently. Therefore, we responded to the calls for caring in these nursing situations in our own unique ways.

Nursing literature and personal research (Kearney, 1991) in caring have enhanced my understanding of caring, which I believe can be expressed in the nursing situation through the nurse's 'way of being,' or personal characteristics, through her presence with the other, and through certain activities or behaviors of the nurse. Let me share some of those ways in which I lived caring with Mrs. Clarke.

My way of being communicated caring in our situation. Mrs. Clarke's courage, openness, and honesty with me called for my being honest, open, and courageous with her. Mayeroff (1971) describes honesty as a positive act of confrontation and being open to oneself and other, rather than a matter of not doing something. Confronting Mrs. Clarke about her smoking and being open with my concerns about her situation conveyed honesty to her. Courage is defined by Mayeroff (1971) as going into the unknown. I demonstrated courage by asking her about her smoking and by choosing not to follow hospital policy. My compassion, or 'kindness,' as she called it, and flexibility with her bath time are other examples of my way of being with her that expressed caring.

Through my presence with Mrs. Clarke, by taking the time to talk and share with her, I lived caring. This notion of spending time with patients is not always understood or valued by nurses. I'll always remember a fellow nurse who spent time with her patients playing cards, watching a ballgame, or even learning to knit. It upset me when I heard other nurses complaining about her wasting time and not 'doing her job.' I now understand that those actions were very much a part of her 'job.' They were an essential part of nursing. She had entered the world of her patients, and was living caring with them in her own unique way. Those special moments may have made an incredible difference in her patients' lives.

I also responded to Mrs. Clarke's call for caring nurturance through my actions. I listened, and encouraged her to express her feelings. I touched her. I provided her with information so that she could make an informed decision, and then, accepted and supported her decision. My nursing responses enhanced her personhood by increasing her understanding of her situation and the risks of her actions, and by nurturing her freedom of choice and confidence in making decisions about how she chose to live her life. My caring enhanced our relationship and possibly future relationships she may have with other nurses and health professionals.

Vicki: Lois' call to remain at home, centered in the familiar activities of daily living clarified my nursing responses to her. I was able to understand that living her life through these rituals supported and nurtured her dignity in dying. The rituals of living daily crossword puzzles with me promoted and enhanced a sense of continuation for her. Superficially, the crossword puzzle ritual might be viewed as a nonnursing activity, but to understand nursing is to know that caring nurturance is engaging in activities which promote personhood.

CONCLUSION

Practicing from this theoretical perspective has guided us in knowing and appreciating our patients more fully. The patients' responses to our caring nurturance have been tremendously rewarding and motivating. We hope our representations of real nursing situations have given the reader a deeper understanding of the beauty of living Nursing As Caring.

REFERENCES

Boykin, A., & Schoenhofer, S. (1993). *The theory of nursing as caring.* New York: National League for Nursing Press.

Kearney, C. (1991). *The patient perspective of caring expressed by nurses through patient explaining (Teaching).* Unpublished Master's Thesis, Florida Atlantic University, Boca Raton, Florida.

Mayeroff, M. (1971). *On caring.* New York: Harper & Row.

Part V

Culture Care Diversity and Universality

9

Culture Care Theory: The Relevant Theory to Guide Nurses Functioning in a Multicultural World

Madeleine Leininger

Nurses are living in a new age of human care services in which they are challenged to know, understand and provide effective care to people of diverse cultures in the world. It is an age in which nurses will have to increase markedly their knowledge and skills as they interact and work with clients from largely unknown cultures during this decade and in the 21st Century. During this time, nurses will face great challenges related to intense multiculturalism as clients expect, demand, and protect their human rights derived from their cultural values, beliefs, and practices. Professional nurses are faced with the challenge to shift from a largely monocultural to a multicultural nursing perspective as nurses work with clients from Eastern Europe, Africa, Australia, Southeast Asia, Oceania, and many places in the world. These challenges are far greater than what nurses have known or experienced today.

Intense multiculturalism will require different approaches and moral obligations to work with clients from different cultures and to deal with uncertainties and transitions. It is, indeed, a world that calls for Culture Care theory to guide them in their work. The theory of Culture Care Diversity and Universality is one of the major relevant and comprehensive theories in nursing which is specifically focused on discovering human care modalities in different cultures in the world (Leininger, 1978, 1991). Culture Care theory has been designed to bring forth new knowledge, insights, and practices about many different or similar cultures in the world. It is one of the oldest nursing theories which began to be developed nearly four decades ago in anticipation that nurses would need a new kind of nursing knowledge to guide their thinking and actions. Accordingly, the theory has provided the broadest and most holistic perspective to study human caring over time and in different places in the world with the goal to develop culturally congruent care derived from specific cultures. Culture Care theory is focused on the *totality of cultural lifeways* with respect to material and non-material cultural care phenomena, but especially care derived from a study of the religion, kinship, political interests, economic views, educational experiences and the world view of different cultures. Specific cultural values, beliefs, and practices related to generic (folk) and professional health care are an integral part of discoveries with the use of the Culture Care theory. Culture Care theory has been the dominant theory to help nurses discover differences and similarities about human care, health, healing, and well being of some of the most unknown and known cultures in the world. Discovering such new insights has brought forth a new revolution as nurses use culturally-based knowledge in learning and serving others. Users of the Culture Care theory have brought forth a new epistemic and ontological base of nursing knowledge with implied moral and ethical expectations for all professional nurses.

In this chapter, some of the major features of the Culture Care theory will be presented, and in the chapter that follows, Kathryn Edmunds applies this theory. The reader must, however, realize that the most complete and definitive works on the theory are found in the published source entitled, *Culture Care Diversity and Universality: A Theory of Nursing* (Leininger, 1991), and in a number of earlier publications focused on the historical evolution and characteristics of the theory covering the past three decades (1970, 1976, 1978, 1981, 1984, 1985, 1988, 1991). In addition, there are a number of nurse researchers, scholars, and students who have been using the theory with different cultures and in different contexts which helps the reader to see the diversity of uses of the theory such as studies by Bohay, 1991; Gates, 1989; Thompson, 1990, and Wenger 1990.

BIRTH, DEVELOPMENT, AND GROWTH OF THE THEORY

It was in the mid-1950s while working as a child mental health clinical specialist that I discovered cultural differences among children. Caring for children of different cultures left me concerned about ways to help them when their behavior expectations and needs were so different. It made me fully aware that I did not have adequate clinical nursing knowledge and skills to care for them. While I could have easily overlooked these cultural differences or labeled them as "strange," "difficult," and "uncooperative," I soon realized that my education and practices in nursing were inadequate regarding cultural factors influencing caring for children of different cultural backgrounds. *Culture* was the big and important missing dimension of nursing and of all health services in the pre-1950s. I was deeply troubled that although nursing had been in existence for nearly 100 years, nurses had not studied, recognized, nor taught about culture factors in nursing education or practice. It became clear to me that nurses could never be effective practitioners or educators in our multicultural world unless they learned about and understood the tremendous importance of cultural beliefs, values, and lifeways of people from different cultures.

Unfortunately, I had never had a course in anthropology nor any instruction about culture, and so I began to remedy this serious deficit by pursuing doctoral study in the field of anthropology as it was the major discipline concerned with diverse cultures in the world and since the beginning of humankind. I soon became the first graduate professional nurse in anthropology. I had worked diligently in the rigorous six year doctoral program studying non-Western and Western cultures. As a part of my educational experiences in anthropology, I soon found myself studying the Gadsup of the Eastern Highlands of New Guinea. It was the Gadsup who taught me that *culture care, health, illness, human birth and development*, were very different from my Anglo-American nursing values, beliefs, and practices learned in nursing in the United States. Practically every day in Gadsup land, I experienced some degree of culture shock and gradually gained new insights about the people and their care values and cultural lifeways. This field experience had a tremendous impact on me and made me aware that nursing education and practices must drastically change to accommodate cultural differences among clients.

After I returned to the United States in the early 1960s, I was convinced that nursing education and practice had to change in all aspects if nursing was to survive and fulfill its societal and worldwide professional expectation of serving human beings worldwide. As a nursing leader, I was committed to change nursing programs so that culture and care phenomena would be included in all aspects of nursing. I remained deeply concerned about the thousands of nurses who were also unaware and unprepared to care for people of different cultures. So upon completion of a rigorous doctoral program in anthropology, I developed undergraduate courses and graduate educational programs in transcultural nursing. This was a major and most formidable task as nurses were mainly interested in the physical and interpersonal needs of patients. Nevertheless, I gradually achieved this goal over the past three decades and almost in a "single-handed" leadership way, until the nurses I prepared took hold and supported the field.

At the same time, I developed my theory of Culture Care and was excited about the theory, for I could envision that all theories and practices needed to include culture with care in nursing. In the late 1940s and in the 1950s, I had identified care as *the central, dominant, and essential component of nursing* (Leininger, 1970, 1978, 1991). I could see that the construct of *culture care* had different meanings, expressions, beliefs, values, and practices with different cultures, and that culture care needed to be studied transculturally. I held and predicted that culture care could be the powerful determinant of health, well-being, and illness patterns of people. Male's and female's behavior was also greatly influenced by culture as well as the ways human beings developed and took on cultural roles and values throughout the life cycle. Culture care patterns and practices were not only important when humans were in good health, but also in death and dying within institutional practices. While continuing to study the theory of Culture Care, I found that care and culture factors were deeply embedded in the world view, social structure, and language uses of a culture. This realization came from my community-based research field observations and documentation which made me aware of the need to study Western and non-Western cultures about human care and wellness patterns.

The theory of Culture Care continued to grow in importance in transcultural nursing and in other areas of nursing. Indeed, after my field research in New Guinea and as the first nurse in transcultural nursing, I was greatly challenged and excited to discover covert care phenomena in New Guinea and felt this discovery was perhaps equally as important as a Nobel Prize winning discovery of a chemical substance. But since this discovery was made using qualitative research methods, it was not recognized as "scientific" because human care in complex cultural structures was not measurable. Nonetheless, I viewed this discovery as a major "breakthrough" with the use of Culture Care theory. It also enabled me to establish a beginning knowledge base for transcultural nursing. Since then the discovery of human care constructs have begun to be incorporated into all nursing education and practice.

The idea of using theories to guide nursing education and practice in the 1950s was unknown or seldom talked about. As I talked about "theory," nurses were not interested in the idea nor did they feel the idea belonged in nursing. I continued, however, to develop and use the theory of Culture Care and to develop the field of transcultural nursing until it all took a firm hold by the mid-1970s. It was actually the graduate nursing students who helped to make Culture Care theory and practices important as a means to improve nursing practices and reduce cultural imposition practices (Leininger, 1989, 1990). Students in the graduate courses in transcultural nursing helped to teach other nurses the importance of the theory and influenced other students, faculty, and clinical nursing staff. It was encouraging to see nursing students committed to the theory and research practices to confront nursing faculty and service personnel about the use of transcultural nursing knowledge in client care.

The theory of Culture Care was enhanced through several lectures on transcultural care in different schools of nursing and health care settings within and outside the United States. I was always pleased and amazed to note that nurses in some countries seemed to respond so quickly to the new idea of transcultural nursing and the theory. Many nurses in Europe and Scandinavia had had considerable experience working with clients of diverse cultures, and they were quick to use the Theory. Besides my many public addresses from 1960 to the present, I published over 160 articles, 24 books and 30 films on the subject of transcultural nursing and culture care. Through the past three decades I remained active with my research using Culture Care and continued to study several Western and non-Western cultures. These leadership efforts, along with the increased numbers of prepared transcultural nurse generalists and specialists in undergraduate and graduate programs, helped Culture Care theory become known worldwide (Leininger, 1991).

Today the nursing theory of *Culture Care Diversity and Universality* is being used in a number of schools of nursing in the United States and overseas. It is being valued for many reasons but especially because it is so relevant to our changing world, with multicultural clients and staff from many places in the world. Some nurses have candidly and enthusiastically said: "It is the only theory that makes sense because it is not only relevant and important in our multicultural world, but because the findings from the theory are so essential and provide guides to good and meaningful client care." Many undergraduate and graduate nursing students have become competent and knowledgeable to use the theory in assessing differences and similarities among clients with respect to their values, beliefs, and practices. The theory has also helped these nurses to realize that culture care factors can make a great difference in providing care to clients, and in their well being and recovery from illness.

Of great importance, the theory has helped nurses to move beyond looking only for physical and emotional "causes" and "diseases" of clients to that of identifying the way culture influences care needs of clients. It has given nurses a fresh approach and different way to understand human beings and their care patterns and needs, and in different contexts, e.g., hospitals, clinics, and workplaces. The theory continues to challenge nurses in exploring some of the most difficult influences such as the impact of religion, family life, music, economics, world views, and other aspects upon caring. The theory has historical significance in that it remains one of the earliest theories in nursing; but one with the longest period of development because the phenomena of culture care was so strange to most nurses, and it was not until nurses were prepared in transcultural nursing that the theory gained meaning and relevance.

ASSUMPTIVE PREMISES OF THE THEORY AND SOME PREDICTIONS

Since the theory of Culture Care was originally conceived in a clinical nursing context and with a deep commitment that *nursing is caring* and culture has an impact on care, the assumptions of the theory were developed with these broad perspectives in mind. The theoretical assumptions were derived, in part, from the use of the ethnonursing and ethnographic qualitative research methods about human care. These factors provided a basis for making assumptions about the theory and for ultimately making interpretations and predictions from the theory. The assumptions about Culture Care served as important broad "givens" and hunches to generate culture care knowledge.

To begin with, I held to the position that *theories served to describe,*

explain, interpret, and provide predictions about the phenomena under study.
This definition was quite different from other nurse researchers who
developed their theories from a logical positivistic perspective with the
goal to get measurable and pre-use outcomes, and to make generaliza-
tions about relationships between different variable or *a priori* hypotheses. Instead, I viewed theories from a naturalistic inquiry mode with
the goal to know, understand, and explain culture care from the people's *emic* (local) views. This qualitative approach in theory use was
essential because there was virtually nothing known about culture care
and its relationship to nursing. A different theory and research approach was imperative to discover culture care.

As the theorist, I pondered about *care* as the central phenomenon
of nursing and *culture* as central to anthropology, and so I wanted to
discover care within a cultural context and study the relationship between culture and care with different cultures and subcultural groups as
well as individuals of particular cultures. In the beginning, I raised several philosophical questions from a nursing and anthropological viewpoint such as: 1) Was *human care* essential to human growth and
survival through the long history of humankind?; 2) What is the relationship between care and culture?; 3) In what ways does culture influence care and caring modes?; 4) How do caring patterns and ways
influence culture?; 5) How might culture care knowledge influence or
change nursing practices in nursing?; 6) If culture care became the substantive and most important base of nursing knowledge, how would
culture care lead to the health and well-being of individuals, families,
groups, cultures, and institutions?; 7) Is human care universal in all cultures?; 8) What might be the power of culture care to advance nursing
care?; 9) Could culture care become a moral ideal or ethical obligation
to nurses? These questions and others led to the assumptions and the
study of culture care phenomenon. While these were exciting questions
to consider, they were also overwhelming to think about. The philosophical questions helped me to formulate the following assumptive
premises about culture care and nursing (Leininger, 1991, pp. 44–45):

1. Care is the essence of nursing and a distinct, dominant, cen-
    tral, and unifying focus.

2. Care (caring) is essential for well-being, health, healing,
    growth, survival, and for facing handicaps or death.

3. Culture care is the broadest holistic means to know, explain, interpret, and predict nursing care phenomena to guide nursing care practices.

4. Nursing is a transcultural humanistic and scientific care discipline and profession, the central purpose of which is to serve human beings worldwide.

5. Care (caring) is essential to curing and healing, for there can be no curing without caring.

6. Culture care concepts, meanings, expressions, patterns, processes, and structural forms of care are different from (diversity) and similar to (toward commonalities or universalities) all cultures of the world.

7. Every human culture has generic (lay, folk, or indigenous) care knowledge and practices, and usually professional care knowledge and practices which vary transculturally.

8. Cultural care values, beliefs, and practices are influenced by and tend to be embedded in the world view, language, religion (or spiritual), kinship (social), political (or legal), educational, economic, technological, ethnohistorical, and environmental contexts of a particular culture.

9. Beneficial, healthy, and satisfying culturally based nursing care contributes to the well-being of individuals, families, groups, and communities within their environmental context.

10. Culturally congruent nursing care can only occur when culture care values, expressions or patterns are known and used appropriately and meaningfully by the nurse with individuals or groups.

11. Culture care differences and similarities between professional care-giver(s) and clients, with their generic needs, exist in human cultures worldwide.

12. Clients who show signs of cultural conflicts, noncompliance, stresses, and ethical or moral concerns, need nursing care that is culturally-based.

13. The qualitative paradigm with naturalistic inquiry modes provides essential means to discover human care transculturally.

These assumptive premises served as a "launching pad" for the study of Culture Care theory and a basis for some predictive hunches.

Since most of nursing instruction, practice, and research had been heavily based upon medical diseases, pathologies, symptoms, and the treatment of diseases, I predicted this could drastically change with a focus on human care as a central phenomenon of nursing. Most importantly, I believed that caring modalities could lead to wellness, health maintenance, and prevention of serious illnesses in the mid-1950s and early 1960s. In fact, I found that prevention of illnesses in New Guinea was based on *protective care* and was stronger than in the United States in those early days. Culture taboos, world views, environmental consideration, and many social structure features regarding kinship rules, spiritual beliefs, and philosophy of life, and culture values were predicted to be a powerful means to prevent illness and remain well through caring expressions and patterns. Interestingly, during my first stay in the two Gadsup villages in the 1960s, there were no psychoses, but at best mild expressions of depression, sexual problems, and intergenerational concerns that could be handled through what I called "culturally-based caring modes."

From my non-Western Gadsup experiences, I was convinced that an inductive *emic* (local viewpoint) was much needed to discover the epistemic and ontologic bases of culture care (Leininger, 1978, 1985). I could see that imposing Western theories, hypotheses, and controlled experiments on humans regarding care would seriously limit the discovery of culture care. Hence, I developed the method and used ethnography for my first culture care study in New Guinea. The ethnonursing method was specifically designed to study the Culture Care theory and I found it so helpful to generate embedded care knowledge that it has been used throughout my research studies along with other qualitative methods such as life histories, visual aids methods, and ethnoscience (Leininger, 1985). Thus, for the first time in the history of nursing, the nursing research method of *ethnonursing* was developed and used to study a nursing theory and nursing phenomenon. The results are noteworthy from the many research findings of nearly 50 cultures (Leininger, 1978, 1984, 1985, 1991).

Through a creative thinking process stimulated by the above philosophical questions and assumptions, the theorist was committed to discover the epistemics and ontologic dimensions of culture care. The theorist held that *care* was the *central, dominant, and unifying focus of nursing.* I predicted that culture care would ultimately offer many rich insights and much new knowledge for the discipline of nursing. I was deeply concerned that human care had been so patently avoided and not studied in nursing except to use the cliché of care and nursing without discovering the meanings and expressions of care, and especially from a transcultural perspective. The statements commonly used in nursing in the 1950s were: "I gave nursing *care* this morning," "This patient needs good nursing *care*"; "*Caring* for this patient has been difficult." What was the meaning of care to nurses and to clients? What constituted care or caring to justify nursing as a discipline and profession? I was always struck by clients who would say: "That nurse gave me wonderful care"; "It was the nurse who cared for me that got me well and out of the hospital." Thus the consumers were aware that nurses who practiced care were instrumental to bring about their health, well being, or healing. However, the meaning of care to American, European, Asian, and all clients in the world was not even considered in nursing in those early days. I, therefore, predicted that culture specific caring actions and processes would lead to health or well being for individuals, families, groups, and cultures. I also predicted that culture care in relation to the client's world view, social structure factors, environmental context, ethnohistory, and language use would lead to the discovery of culture care phenomenon that had never been known to nurses. The way that religion, kinship ties, economics, political forces, educational modes and technologies influenced care patterns was important to me, as well as the environmental context and ethnohistorical accounts of clients.

Most importantly, I predicted that there would be care structures, patterns, meanings, forms of expressions, and practices that would be different transculturally and these would be the cultural diversities of culture care. At the same time, I predicted there would be some universal features, patterns, and expressions of care over time and in different places in the world. These commonalities about care would be, in time, the universal knowledge to guide nurses in giving culturally congruent care. They would also help nurses to feel united in some common care constructs one could rely upon in all areas of nursing. I did not conceive of culture care from an absolute view, but more from commonalities or predominant themes about *homo sapiens* transculturally. If knowledge could be discovered, it would provide the epistemic and ontologic dimension of nursing knowledge as diversities or universalities.

Nursing might some day in the 21st Century have a wealth of care knowledge to teach and guide nursing practice. This would move nursing from dependence on medical activities. I coined the term *culture specific* and *culture congruent care* to help nurses realize that all cultures could be served with these ideas in mind.

In conceptualizing the theory of Culture Care, I not only predicted that world view, social structure, ethnohistory, and environment would have an influence on culture care expressions and patterns, but that these influences would explain and predict the health or well being of people. I also predicted that *generic* or *folk* care and *professional* care would reveal diversities and influence nursing care outcomes related to whether one could provide culturally congruent care. Finally, I predicted three nursing decision or action modes, namely: 1) *Cultural care preservation/maintenance*; 2) *Cultural care accommodation/negotiation*; and 3) *Cultural care repatterning and restructuring* (Leininger, 1991, pp. 41–42). If data were used from the above prediction areas, i.e., world view, social structure, environment, generic and professional health systems, it would guide nurses to use the appropriate nursing care mode(s) to provide culturally congruent care. Other specifics of the theory are discussed in my recent definitive work (Leininger, 1991) and will not be repeated here.

In sum, the *purpose* of the theory was to discover knowledge about culture care diversities and universalities and to use this knowledge to guide, improve, or provide new kinds of nursing care. The goal of the theory was to describe, understand, and predict culture care that was meaningful, beneficial, and healing to individuals, families, groups, cultures, and even institutions with *culturally congruent nursing care practices*. I held that if care was not culturally congruent or appropriate, it would have unfavorable consequences, or would be rejected by clients because the care did not reasonably fit the cultural values, beliefs, and lifeways of those being cared for or about. Moreover, one could predict legal suits and many unfavorable outcomes. In addition, clients from some cultures would not use health care systems that were not congruent with their beliefs and lifeways.

ORIENTATIONAL DEFINITIONS

Since the research discovery method of ethnonursing to study Culture Care theory was developed within the qualitative paradigm, orientational definitions were used as guides to study culture care phenomena. These definitions were as follows (Leininger, 1991, pp. 46–49).

1. *Care* (noun) refers to abstract and concrete phenomena related to assisting, supporting or enabling experiences or behaviors toward or for others, with evident or anticipated needs to ameliorate or improve a human condition or lifeway.

2. *Caring* (gerund) refers to actions or activities directed toward assisting, supporting, or enabling another individual or group with evident or anticipated needs, to ameliorate or improve a human condition or lifeway, or to face death.

3. *Culture* refers to the learned, shared, and transmitted values, beliefs, norms, and lifeways of a particular group that guides their thinking, decisions, and actions in patterned ways.

4. *Cultural care* refers to the cognitively learned and transmitted values, beliefs, and patterned lifeways that tend to assist, support, or enable another individual or group to maintain their well-being, health, or to improve their human condition and lifeways, or to deal with illness, handicaps, or death.

5. *Culture care diversity* refers to the variabilities or differences in meanings, patterns, values, lifeways or symbols of care within or between collectivities that are related to assistive, supportive, or enabling human care expressions.

6. *Culture care universality* refers to the common, similar, or dominant uniform care meanings, patterns, values, or symbols that are manifest among many cultures which reflect assistive, supportive, or enabling ways to help people. (Universality is not used as an absolute nor a statistically significant referent.)

7. *Nursing* refers to a learned humanistic and scientific profession and discipline which is focused on human care phenomena and activities in order to assist, support, enable or facilitate individuals or groups to maintain or regain their well-being (or health) in culturally meaningful and beneficial ways, or to help individuals face death.

8. *World view* refers to the way people tend to look out upon the world or their universe to form a picture or a value stance about their life or world around them.

9. *Cultural and social structure dimensions* refers to the dynamic patterns and features of interrelated structural and organizational factors of a particular culture (subculture or society) which includes religious, kinship (social), political, economic, educational, technologic, and cultural values, and how these factors function and influence human behavior in different environmental contexts.

10. *Environmental context* refers to the totality of an event, situation, or particular experience that gives meaning to human expressions, interpretations, and social interactions in particular physical, ecological, and cultural settings.

11. *Ethnohistory* refers to those past facts, events, instances, experiences of individuals, groups, cultures and institutions that are primarily people (ethno) centered and which describe, explain, and interpret human lifeways within cultural contexts.

12. *Generic folk or lay system* refers to culturally learned and transmitted lay, indigenous (traditional), or folk (home care) knowledge and skills used to provide assistive, supportive, enabling, or facilitative acts (or phenomena) toward or for another individual, group or institution with evident or anticipated needs to ameliorate or improve a human health condition (or well-being), disability, lifeway, or to face death.

13. *Professional system* refers to formal and cognitively learned professional care knowledge and practice skills that are used to provide assistive, supportive, enabling or facilitative acts, to or for another individual or group in order to improve a human health condition (or well-being), disability, lifeway, or to work with dying clients.

14. *Health* refers to a state of well-being that is culturally defined, valued, and practiced, and which reflects the ability of individuals (or groups) to perform their daily role activities in culturally expressed, beneficial, and patterned ways.

15. *Culture care preservation or maintenance* refers to those assist-ive, supporting, or enabling professional actions and deci-sions that help people of a particular culture retain or preserve relevant care values that help them maintain their well-being or recover from illness, or to face handicaps or death.

16. *Culture care accommodation or negotiation* refers to those as-sistive, supporting, or enabling creative professional actions and decisions that help a client(s) or a designated culture adapt to or negotiate for a beneficial or satisfying health out-come with professional care-providers.

17. *Culture care repatterning or restructuring* refers to those assist-ive, supporting, or enabling professional actions and deci-sions that help a client(s) reorder, change, or modify their lifeways for new or different health care patterns, and which respect their cultural values and beliefs as well as provide a healthier life pattern.

18. *Culture congruent (nursing) care* refers to those assistive, sup-portive, or enabling acts that fit with the cultural values, beliefs, and lifeways of a client, group, culture, community, or institution; in meaningful, beneficial, or satisfying ways, and which result in positive outcomes.

THE SUNRISE MODEL TO DEPICT THE THEORY

Within the assumptive premises, theoretical predictions, and orienta-tional constructs, the Sunrise Model (Figure 9.1) was used to guide nurses in visualizing the different dimensions of the theory with direc-tional influences on cultural care expressions and patterns, and with a focus on the three predicted modes of nursing actions. This model or cognitive map, is used to orient nurses to care influences, rather than as a conceptual framework *per se*. It is important in using this model to keep in mind the different care influences with thought to how findings from these influences can lead to providing culturally congruent care as the goal of the theory.

Although the theory was developed primarily to generate *emic*, or grounded substantive data about culture care meanings, patterns and

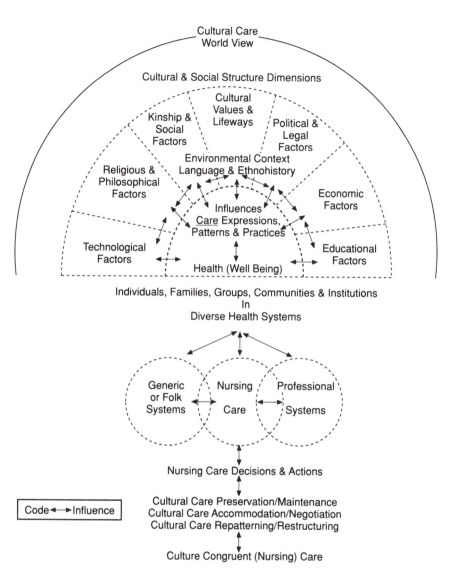

Reprinted from *Culture Care Diversity and Universality: A Theory of Nursing*, Madeline M.
Leininger, editor (1991). Published by National League for Nursing Press.

Figure 9.1 Leininger's Sunrise Model to depict Theory of Cultural Care Diversity and Universality.

experiences of informants from data gathered using the Sunrise Model, the theory could be used within the quantitative paradigm. I would predict, however, that the findings would need data from the qualitative paradigm to have meaning, relevance and credibility because human care cannot be readily measured and controlled. It is also important to note that all the data generated within the qualitative paradigm were analyzed using qualitative criteria such as credibility, meaning-in-context, recurrent patterning, saturation (and redundancy), and confirmability (Leininger, 1991).

Currently, the theory of Culture Care is rapidly growing in its use within nursing and other disciplines. The demand for the theory is largely due to: 1) the rich and meaningful data being generated from culture care studies; 2) the high relevance of findings to improve client care; 3) the holistic focus of the theory; 4) the fact that the theory has both abstract and very practical features; 5) explication of detailed meanings of care and uses for congruent care; 6) diverse foci on cultures, families, individuals, institutions, and groups; 7) the great learning opportunities for the researcher to gain knowledge, especially about cultures; 8) the positive feedback from informants about the research focus in care as "useful and relevant"; 9) the fact that informants liked the research approach and methods. The theory is also being used today to study nursing administration and corporate hospital structures.

In general, the theory of Culture Care will continue to grow in use worldwide because it is not culture-bound, and is open to discover data which has not previously been known, or has been vaguely known. The theory is also open for creative formulations related to the domain of culture care and its predicted influence on health or well-being. This feature also makes the theory attractive to many nurses and others interested in discovering culture care phenomenon and using the findings in appropriate ways to improve a human condition or lifeway. I predict the theory findings will have a significant impact on nursing and health care and will also be used by many disciplines in the future.

REFERENCES

Leininger, M. (1970). *Nursing and anthropology: Two worlds to blend.* New York: John Wiley & Sons.

Leininger, M. (1976). Caring: The essence and central focus of nursing. American Nurses Foundation. *Nursing Research Report*, 12(1), 2, 14.

Leininger, M. (1978). *Transcultural nursing: Concepts, theories, and practices.* New York: John Wiley & Sons.

Leininger, M. (1981). *Care: An essential human need.* Thorofare, NJ: Slack.

Leininger, M. (1984). *Care: The essence of nursing and health.* Thorofare, NJ: Slack.

Leininger, M. (1985). Qualitative research methods in nursing (pp. 33–73). Orlando, FL: Grune and Stratton Company.

Leininger, M. (1988). Leininger's Theory of Nursing: Culture Care Diversity and Universality. *Nursing Science Quarterly*, Vol. 2, No. 4, 11–20. Baltimore, MD: Williams & Wilkins Press.

Leininger, M. (1990b). Ethnomethods: The philosophic and epistemic basis to explicate transcultural nursing knowledge. *Journal of Transcultural Nursing*, Vol. 1, No. 2, Winter issue, 40–51.

Leininger, M. (1991). *Culture care diversity and universality: A theory of Nursing.* New York: National League for Nursing Press.

10

Transcultural Nursing Care with Old Colony Mennonites in a School Context

Kathryn Edmunds

The purpose of Leininger's theory of Culture Care Diversity and Universality is to discover knowledge and gain understanding, and to use the knowledge purposefully to give effective and meaningful nursing care to people (Leininger, 1985a, 1988, 1991). The theory provides a holistic means to discover cultural care that can be assessed, described, interpreted and predicted. Leininger defines cultural care as the "subjectively and objectively learned and transmitted values, beliefs and patterned lifeways that assist, support, facilitate, or enable another individual or group to maintain their well-being, health, to improve their human condition and lifeway, or to deal with illness, handicaps, or death" (1991, p. 47). Leininger's theoretical assumptions, definitions, and predictive hunches were used in this study as presented in Chapter Nine.

This chapter will show how the theory of Culture Care was used with theoretical research questions to explicate and study the Old Colony Mennonite culture. The ethnonursing research method was used to generate culturally congruent care knowledge as a basis for nursing decisions or actions. Leininger's Sunrise Model, (p. 119) as a cognitive map, was used to explore broad and yet specific cultural care factors held to influence the health or well-being of people. Dimensions such as world view, ethnohistory, cultural and social structure, environmental context, language, and professional and generic health structures are systematically examined. Culturally congruent nursing care decisions and actions for Old Colony Mennonites were predicted to be the goal of the theory.

RESEARCHER'S INTEREST

My initial interest in studying this culture arose in my practice as a public health nurse in a rural area of Southwestern Ontario, Canada, and with graduate preparation in the field of transcultural nursing. While enrolled in the transcultural nursing program, I began to realize that my nursing care was not culturally appropriate and I was handicapped to give total or quality care.[1] I did not have the knowledge nor understanding to plan for effective and culturally competent nursing actions. I began to study anthropological and sociological literature and discovered several excellent references of Old Colony Mennonite history (Redekop, 1969; Sawatzky, 1971). There were, however, no studies which examined health or care practices specific to this culture. Culture Care theory helped me to discover the larger picture of human lifeways and to gain insights about the care values, meanings and practices of specific cultures. This was invaluable and essential to broadening my outlook considerably to comprehend new perspectives of the Mennonite culture and their lifeways. It was a new and different challenge to my thinking and research.

RESEARCH QUESTIONS

The ethnonursing research method was designed by Leininger (1985b, 1991) specifically for the systematic study of the Culture Care theory. It was a tailor-made method to study the domain of inquiry which was focused on the explication of Old Colony Mennonite maternal-child care values and practices.

The following research questions were developed as a general guide to study the domain within Leininger's Culture Care theory:

---

[1] In keeping with the ethnonursing qualitative research method, I will be using the first and third person referent to reflect direct participatory lived experiences.

1. What are the specific cultural care meanings, beliefs and practices related to maternal-child health of Old Colony Mennonites?

2. What cultural and social structure dimensions influence their maternal-child caring lifeways and health practices?

3. In light of Old Colony Mennonite traditional and current care practices, how is the health or well being of the women and young children influenced?

4. What theoretical and practice implications can be drawn from the ethnonursing data to generate culturally congruent nursing decisions or actions with the Old Colony Mennonites?

RESEARCH METHOD AND ENTERING THE MENNONITE WORLD

The ethnonursing research method has been described in other sources to which readers are referred (Leininger, 1985b, 1991). I used Leininger's Cultural Care and Health Lifestyle Interview guide with open-ended questions that focused on maternal-child health and care practices. Leininger's guide, called the *Ethnonursing Observation-Participation-Reflection Phases* (1991) was helpful in the research process in order to obtain *emic* detailed data. I conducted the ethnonursing study in the people's familiar environment. Since the informants were all born and had lived in Old Colony settlements in Mexico and had migrated to Southwestern Ontario, the study was conducted in the latter location. The interviews took place in the informant's natural and familiar home setting. I had two key and five general informants who were purposefully chosen because of their in-depth knowledge of the culture and willingness to share information with me for the study. I visited with the key informants for 2 to 3 hours and with general informants for a shorter time of approximately 45 minutes to 1 hour.

When using the ethnonursing method, the researcher begins the first day to observe, document, and analyze data. Documentation consisted of a field work journal and condensed and expanded accounts of observations and interviews. Data analysis was continuous. Leininger's *Four Phases of Ethnonursing Analysis of Qualitative Data* (1991) was used to identify care values, meanings, and patterns.

Since my nursing practice was focused in Canadian schools, I requested to be assigned to an Old Colony Mennonite private school when it opened in 1990. I had begun the ethnonursing research with this culture and wanted to study the theory and apply my knowledge to a practice setting which the method facilitated. Classes on puberty, reproduction, and decision-making were a part of the public school curriculum but were not taught at the Old Colony school. I offered these classes to the Old Colony Mennonite teachers and was invited by the Mennonite School board to attend a parents meeting to discuss the content and structure of potential presentations to the students. I was very concerned about the appropriate way to explore this subject because it was a sensitive issue due to their religious beliefs and practices. However, as a transcultural nurse, my mentor had emphasized the use of the Culture Care theory and a culturalogical assessment with the Sunrise Model to derive insight of how best to proceed. In this chapter, I will first show the theoretical components and data discovered, followed by nursing care actions and decisions that are derived from the ethnonursing research method and the theory data. The practical aspects of the theory findings for planning and implementing of the classes will be discussed in light of the three modes of action and decision related to the theory in order to provide culture congruent and meaningful care.

ETHNOHISTORY

The ethnohistory of Old Colony Mennonites was very interesting and became a major guide for understanding the people and developing data bearing upon the theory and transcultural nursing. The Mennonites were a part of the Anabaptist movement which emerged during the Protestant Reformation in Europe in the early 16th century (Epp, 1974). In 1529 Anabaptism was declared illegal and its followers were persecuted. Nevertheless, the movement spread throughout Northern Europe and in 1536, Menno Simmons, a Dutch Catholic priest, renounced Catholicism and was baptized in the new faith. Through his writings and leadership at a crucial time, Mennonites became distinct from other Anabaptists. Basic tenets of the faith centered on the complete separation of church and state, confession of faith by believers prior to baptism (i.e., adult baptism), Christian obedience and non-resistance to violence, and the belief in preaching the word of God as central to religious experience (N. N. Driedger, 1972).

Old Colony Mennonites have had several major migrations in search of religious freedom and government non-interference in their way of life. In Prussia, Low German was adopted as the oral language; High German became the written language and was used during religious services (Friesen, 1988). The first Mennonite families who arrived in Russia founded the colony of Chortitza in 1789, and since this was the first Russian settlement it became known as the "old colony" (N. N. Driedger, 1972). Old Colony Mennonites today are descendants of the people who lived in Chortitza. According to Epp (1974), between 1874–1880, when Russia introduced compulsory conscription and promoted cultural integration of settlers, one third of all Russian Mennonites left for Canada and the United States. There were 7,000 Mennonites who settled in Manitoba, Canada. They were more conservative and believed that non-resistance and preservation of their culture were of great importance (Epp, 1974).

The precipitating factor of the next migration from Canada to Mexico was related to the desire to educate their children according to their religious and cultural beliefs. The Manitoba Public Schools Act of 1890 abolished tax support for denominational schools, but this Act was not enforced until after World War I. Enforcement came in a climate of postwar militarism and anti-German sentiment with inspectors visiting the Old Colony Mennonite schools and imposing many fines for use of the Mennonite curriculum (Epp, 1982). Conservative Mennonite congregations found it was an intolerable intrusion of their right to educate their children in their own schools using the German language and according to their cultural and religious traditions.

The response of the Old Colony Mennonites to government intervention was already established by previous migrations. It was one of resistance, withdrawal and yet another migration in order to preserve their way of life. Between 1922 and 1926, H. L. Sawatzky (1971, p. 64) identified that 6,000 Mennonites moved to Mexico to begin anew the work of clearing the land and forming villages. Due to the large number of children per family, the Mennonite population in Mexico had increased to 50,000 in 1987 (Warkentin, 1987, p. 2). Since then, land holdings have not increased to the same extent as population growth; this led to a landless population of approximately 30 percent.

Overcrowding of the colonies in Mexico and deteriorating economic conditions in that country led to migration back to Canada.

Some Old Colony Mennonites returned to Manitoba, but even greater numbers came to Southwestern Ontario (where there was no original settlement) due to the need for agricultural laborers. The first few Mennonite families from Mexico arrived in Southwestern Ontario twenty-five to thirty years ago and immigration has since increased. It is estimated by the Mennonite Central Committee that there are currently 15–17,000 Mennonites from Mexico in southern Ontario (Dueck, 1989, p. 2). While all previous migrations occurred in response to perceived or real threats to Old Colony religious and cultural values, this most recent migration to Canada was based on more economic than religious reasons. The migration was not planned by the leadership of the colonies in Mexico and it continues to occur. This synopsis of the ethnohistory reveals the dispersed patterns of migration and the perception by Old Colony Mennonites that outsiders were considered as non-caring as they searched for religious freedom and economic and cultural isolation. Deprivations experienced during migrations had a negative impact on health and well being.

CULTURAL AND SOCIAL STRUCTURE DIMENSIONS

World View

The world view of cultures provided the viewpoint of the people as they looked out on the world about them. It is an important area of knowledge to examine dimensions of the theory of Culture Care. The world view of Old Colony Mennonites was characterized as being a closed community separate and apart from "the world." They saw themselves as the "children of Israel" facing migration and persecution in order to be true to the word of God (Redekop, 1969). Because worldly contact was seen as sinful and offering temptations that must be resisted, contact with outside groups (including other Mennonites) had negative connotations. Their world view of each other was one of *closeness* and *presence* which was evident in the daily life in the Old Colony Mennonite community and reinforced by their religious beliefs.

Religious and Philosophical Factors

Studying the religious and philosophical factors influencing Old Colony Mennonites, it became clear that they believed they were God's chosen people. Salvation was not personal but collective; God would take care of those who were faithful and punish those who did not remain pure from the world (Redekop, 1969). A basic tenet of Anabaptism was the separation of church and state so that the church could remain "pure." However, within Old Colony society, the religious and secular life of members of the congregation (*Gemeinde*) could not be separated (L. Driedger, 1988). Fragmentation and dependence on one's congregation had also been a part of the general Anabaptist movement as there had been no central authority or institution for all Mennonites (Epp, 1982). Differing opinions of biblical interpretation, past persecution and migration led to maintained fragmentation of the Mennonite community. Even among Old Colony congregations differences exist which have prohibited them from proselytizing. There has been no history of welcoming potential converts. The culture supported endogamy (marry with the community), and so members were kept within the Old Colony context supported by their beliefs and traditions.

Led by their bishops and elders, congregational decisions have been biblically based (Epp, 1982). The roles, behavior and dress of women and men are also based on scriptural interpretation. Husbands are the head of the family as part of the proper relationship between men and women. Dress for both sexes was modest and plain, and so jewelry and cosmetics were not worn, as it would be sinful to take undue pride in one's appearance. Married Old Colony women wore head coverings at all times as symbols of their status in the community and in order to pray. This was an extension of the biblical injunction that women should have their hair covered while at worship (Horst, 1934). Marriage and children were viewed as part of God's plan for all members of the community. Birth control was not sanctioned as children are a blessing from God. Interfering with child bearing would be going against God's will.

Church services are an important part of community life. Ministers are elected by the congregation from one of their (male) members and are expected to preach from books of prepared sermons that are passed on from previous ministers. Men and women sit on opposite sides of the church. The church had virtually no pictures or displays of wealth which reflected the values of a modest and non-materialistic lifeway.

Religion was an essential factor in the lives of the families interviewed. One woman said "When you are baptized it ties the knot with God. You try and live as He would want." Another woman stated "If a person is unreligious—why should they care about the next person?"

When asked to describe their daily routines all responded: "The first thing we do is pray." Thus religion played a central and major role in relation to health and well being. Care was expressed by being a religious person and following the word of God. Without spiritual relatedness, the people perceived there would be no reason to care. Lack of spiritual relatedness was also perceived to have a negative impact on well-being.

Kinship, Social and Cultural Factors

According to biblical beliefs, the family remains the foundation of Old Colony social structure. The kinship structure was patrilineal and patriarchal which governed the family lifeway (Sawatzky, 1971). Fathers were the head of the household and provided for the family in material and spiritual ways. Mothers were responsible for the home and children. Grandparents were respected as givers of advice based on the knowledge of life experiences. Children were taught to obey and respect their parents and other adults. Conformity to community norms was essential and highly valued as opposed to individual expressions of dissent or self-determination (Redekop, 1969). Rules of conduct were stretched more for men than for women. For example, smoking or drinking alcohol was acceptable for men by virtue of their superior authority.

The main kinship activity of the culture in Canada was visiting. It was important to keep in contact with relatives who are visited as often as time and distance will allow. Children are expected to visit with the family. Contact was also kept through letter writing. Letters are mailed directly or sent to a newspaper published in Manitoba which is then mailed throughout South and Central America. The author found that mutual aid as practiced by the Old Colony community was more limited than among the Old Order Amish as described by Wenger and Wenger (1988). The Old Colony *Gemeinde* may provide limited help in times of adversity, but families are expected to provide for themselves. Within families, mutual aid remained valued and relatives in Canada and Mexico were assisted as much as possible.

Cultural values and care expressions related to well-being were discussed by Old Colony Mennonites as being extremely important. Care expressions were grounded in religious beliefs and practices and were demonstrated as *respect for tradition* and *being responsible for children*. Being connected to a community with a shared history and current traditions was also important for well being and health. For women, carrying on the traditions of dress, especially the head covering and saying prayers were seen as being important parts of Old Colony culture as well as statements of religious belief. Husbands and wives say prayers before rising and at night. Children are included in family praying before and after meals. As one informant stated, "My mother taught me to keep up my home; the children and religion were the way they were taught, and to never forget my prayers."

Educational Factors

It is difficult to underestimate the impact of education as it has been defined and valued by Old Colony Mennonites. Education was embedded in the cultural values and religious beliefs. It was always considered to be important prior to migration to Canada or to Mexico. The philosophy of education has been that the schools were expected to supplement learning in the home. Children learned the skills they needed in the home and about agriculture from their parents. The purpose of formal education had been traditionally to provide basic reading and writing skills and religious instruction in the German language (Epp, 1982).

As stated earlier, disputes over educational standards and control led to the migration from Manitoba to Mexico. Not only did Old Colony Mennonites feel strongly that their way of life was being threatened by association with the outer "world" of the Canadian school system, but the attempted imposition of a culturally inappropriate educational system created a cultural backlash which is still of concern to the people. Formal education and changes to the existing system have been viewed wlth suspicion by the Old Colony Mennonite clergy in Mexico who have direct control of the schools (Sawatzky, 1971). Children attend school from the ages of seven to twelve or thirteen where learning occurs based on rote learning, rather than the natural or creative expression or synthesis of children's ideas. In 1971, Sawatzky (p. 305) estimated that 90 percent of Mennonites in Mexico were below functional literacy. An informant who had been educated in Mexico commented, "What they learn here [in Canada] is so different. I had only four years of school, then I was at home and on the farm." She added, "High school education does not look promising. They don't need all that education."

The oral language of Old Colony Mennonites was based on 17th century West Prussian Platt or Plaudietsch (Friesen, 1988), which was distinct from present day German with no written expression. German business language from the 18th century had been used for writing and had remained essentially the same since its adoption by Old Colony Mennonites. Revisions and additions to the language and the school system in Mexico have been resisted in order to protect cultural integrity and separation from the world. Concern for the well being of children had been expressed by community involvement in the private school system which valued and respected the traditions of religion, a shared history apart from the world, and kinship ties.

In Southwestern Ontario, the Old Colony Mennonite Church founded a private school in 1990. Initial enrollment was higher than expected and the school was seen as a positive development by the Old Colony community. Grades one through twelve are offered and classes taught in English, with prayers and hymns in German. Providing a private Old Colony Mennonite education to their children was perceived as being a parental obligation and a caring response in order to preserve religious and cultural values.

Technological Factors

The traditional lifestyle of Old Colony Mennonites has been and remains agrarian. It was based and maintained on both individual incentives and community self-sufficiency (Sawatzky, 1971). In the area of agriculture, technological advances have been accepted, though older equipment was used to avoid being too modern. After the Mennonites arrived in Mexico, they discovered the soil was poorer in quality than in Canada or Russia. They experimented with different crops and growing methods (Sawatzky, 1971). Used tractors and other farm machinery were imported to Mexico from the United States. Generators were used to provide electricity to the machine shop and the barn but not in the home. Electricity in the home was not used to avoid bringing the world inside.

Health care technologies have been accepted by Old Colony Mennonites. While the folk health system remains valued, the researcher found there were no sanctions against receiving professional medical treatment or services that would require laboratory tests, surgery, or anaesthetics. Drugs that were dispensed by prescription in Canada were readily available in Mexico on an "over-the-counter" basis. Most families stated that these medications were purchased and administered (often by injection) by the father or mother in a household.

Today in Mexico, modern tractors and cars are used more frequently than in the past. This has led to increased contact with other Mennonite settlements and with Mexicans. Among current technologies are cars, radios, tractors, and electricity; whose use is frequently debated and discussed with respect to modernity. While technology is used, it has more limited value related to technological practices and care modes of community members. Technology is used mainly for agricultural production and distribution. In Southwestern Ontario most Old Colony Mennonite families had electricity in their homes and a car. Currently, the same debate exists in Canada and Mexico as local congregations struggle to find a balance between technological benefits, increased exposure to the world, and religious expectations of salvation that promote isolation.

Economic Factors

The Old Colony Mennonites have been dependent upon agriculture as their subsistence and current economic base. The land was valued and enabled the community to be self-sustaining and independent from the rest of the world. Land ownership by families rather than by the community had characterized traditional Old Colony settlements (Sawatzky, 1971). When migrations occurred, families would purchase equal amounts of land and subsequent generations would follow this practice. Increase in the amount of land owned by Mennonites in Mexico has not kept pace with the sevenfold increase in population (Warkentin, 1987). This has led to a class distinction between the landowners (Worte) and the landless (Anwohner). Even though land was family owned through the fathers, the traditional belief existed that all families were equal members of the congregation. The large number of landless in Mexico today was a new development in Old Colony history and a class structure has emerged which has caused further divisions in the community.

Inflation, deteriorating economic conditions, and lack of land ownership have contributed to the financial destitution of many Old Colony Mennonites in Mexico. This has led to the current migration from Mexico back to Canada. Salaries for agricultural work were higher in Canada and services such as social assistance and unemployment insurance were available. Family care modalities related to kinship and role responsibilities were evident in agricultural work and in showing the interdependence of families.

Political and Legal Factors

Mennonites have traditionally been opposed to the swearing of oaths (N. N. Driedger, 1972) as part of their belief in the separation of church and state and noninvolvement in government. Affirmations were given instead and this practice continues today. Accordingly, Old Colony Mennonites were not politically involved in agencies such as the town council, public school board, and community centers. One woman interviewed stated "prayer alone will guide others to do the right thing." The grandparents and greatgrandparents of today's young adults were Canadian citizens. In many cases, Mennonites migrating from Mexico to Canada were eligible for Canadian citizenship. Those Old Colony Mennonites who arrived in Canada and could speak English were usually not viewed as literate. Therefore, confusion regarding forms for legal status and eligibility for social programs was common. There were no religious sanctions against receiving government assistance. The Mennonite Central Committee office provided help in completing forms and applications. There was also an informal network where family members who are able to communicate in English and are familiar with the Canadian system would express care through mutual aid by accompanying people to appointments or hearings.

The role of the Old Colony Mennonite Church in political and legal matters was limited and reinforced the value of cultural isolation. However, the church does reinforce community activities and provided protective care pertaining to religion, culture, and education. Some Old Colony families migrated to Canada and retained affiliation with their congregation in Mexico. This isolated them from church protective care while in Canada.

GENERIC (FOLK) AND PROFESSIONAL NURSING FACTORS

Because of the educational values, the researcher found there were no formally trained traditional Old Colony health practitioners. However, generic or folk health practices within the Old Colony Mennonite community existed. In Mexico, lay pharmacists, chiropractors, and midwives were openly consulted. One informant stated, "In Mexico, you go to the pharmacist. You tell him what's wrong and he will figure out what you need." Another informant related, "My husband has the touch to set bones, just like his father and grandfather. . . . He knows by touch what to do." Midwives were used to "reposition" the fetus during pregnancy to facilitate an easier labor and delivery. The generic system was used for 'everyday' concerns and preventive services.

Access to the professional health care system in Mexico was based on the ability to pay. Financial constraints and negative experiences with health care institutions such as the perception of a poor quality of service have limited use of the professional health care system. Routine consultation with physicians for preventative or health promotion services did not occur. Public health nursing services were often limited to sporadic immunization programs.

In Canada, the professional health care system may be reluctantly used by Old Colony Mennonites because of past experiences in Mexico. This is sometimes interpreted by professionals as placing a low value on disease prevention and health promotion, for example, non-attendance at prenatal visits to a physician in which the client may then be described as "non-compliant." Many Canadian professional health care providers are not aware of the historical and cultural reasons for behavior such as missing prenatal appointments and therefore negatively label what is not understood. Nevertheless, Old Colony Mennonites do use the government funded Canadian health care system. Public health nurses are accepted in their homes and families are receptive to health teaching when it is done in a culturally sensitive way. Physicians are consulted and deliveries take place in hospitals. Alongside the professional system and largely unknown by it, the generic health system continues to exist.

CARE MEANINGS AND PATTERNS

Old Colony Mennonite care values and practices centered on their religion, culture, traditions, and responsibilities toward children. Health occurs when a person engages in age and sex-appropriate activities and leads their life "as God would want." Healthy lifeways involve eating "good" foods, avoiding physical overexertion, and the use of prayer.

There are no formal ceremonies or rituals associated with puberty, pregnancy or childbirth. Puberty and reproduction are very private matters and any teaching is done by the same-sex parent. Young women usually have very little knowledge about reproductive physiology and if any information is given, it is not until the age of fourteen or older. Pregnancies are not discussed with other children in the family. The dominant culture care meanings and action patterns were: (1) *presence*, especially of family members (for example, extended families or mothers with their children); (2) *spiritual relatedness*, such as the use of prayer in daily routines and during times of physical or emotional stress; (3) *being responsible for*, especially mothers toward children; (4) *respect for traditional lifeways and values*; (5) *reciprocity* (for example, mutual aid among families); (6) *connectedness* with extended family members, the community and a shared history; and (7) *privacy* related to sexual matters.

These care meanings were embedded in the Old Colony Mennonite world view and social structure dimensions which had a significant influence on care patterns, health, and well being. The most important factors identified for influencing care and health were: (1) world view; (2) religious and philosophical beliefs; (3) kinship, social and cultural factors; (4) educational factors and (5) economic way of life as an agrarian society.

The world view and religious beliefs and practices were powerful influences on human caring. Religious and cultural isolation reinforced the meaning of care as being responsible for others in the community, present, connected to a shared history, and spiritually related to God. Isolation also produced a rich generic health care system for illness and preventive care practices. While treatment and technology used by the professional health care system have been accepted, Old Colony Mennonite families may be unaware of many procedures, practices, and assumptions used by health professionals. Attempts to provide care by nurses and other professionals may be distrusted.

Traditional Old Colony communities are no longer immune from changes occurring in the societies in which they live (L. Driedger, 1986). Economic divisions, religious debates, and migration have increased community and family fragmentation. Resistance to change was evident through caring behaviors which show respect for religious, cultural, and kinship traditions. Mutual aid continues to be practiced and families place a high value on traditional kinship care patterns.

Education and language also have a major influence on health in that professional health education was not part of the traditional curriculum. Care meanings of respect for educational traditions and privacy may have a negative effect on health and well-being if health care assessments and culturally appropriate interventions are delayed due to the language barrier, reluctance to discuss private concerns, or lack of knowledge.

NURSING CARE DECISIONS AND ACTIONS

Leininger's Culture Care theory predicts that culturally congruent nursing care based on assessment of social structure, values and lifeways will provide nursing care that is "meaningful, satisfying and beneficial care to clients" (1988, p. 155). The researcher identified several transcultural guidelines for providing culture congruent care. First, prior planning and reflection was an important component of this process. Access to teach classes on puberty in the school needed to be planned and implemented through parents. Intergenerational differences existed, which was important for the transcultural nurse to recognize and respect. For example, the parents who had been born and had attended traditional schools in Mexico, had different expectations in care. Many of their children had been born in Canada and had attended public schools where they would have been exposed to a much broader and varied life experience. Leininger's (1985b, 1991) *Stranger to Trusted Friend Enabler Guide* was also helpful in planning nursing care. The parents did not know me as well as the students or the teachers so I was able to anticipate a somewhat guarded response. The parents, however, showed gradual signs of trusting me as a friend and someone sensitive to them on the difficult topic.

Drawing upon research findings from world view, social structure, language, generic (folk) and professional health care, Leininger's three modes of nursing actions and decisions were identified and used to provide culture congruent care. They will be discussed next.

I.   **Culture care preservation or maintenance** "refers to those assistive, supporting, facilitative, or enabling professional actions and decisions that help people of a particular culture to retain and/or preserve relevant care values so that they can maintain their well being, recover from illness, or face handicaps and/or death" (Leininger, 1991, p. 48). The researcher used the care concepts of respect and presence as a way to preserve Old Colony Mennonite religious values. My remarks to the parents were prefaced by stating that what I would say to them and what I would teach their children was based on respect for oneself and respect for others. I recognized that the parents were demonstrating concern for their children's health through their presence with each other and by using prayer at the meeting.

Language used in the presentation to the parents was general and not detailed. This was done for two reasons (1) English was their second language and (2) my knowledge that matters pertaining to sexual development are traditionally very private and not openly discussed in mixed groups meant that to specifically discuss topics in detail could have been embarrassing and possibly offensive. I provided culture care preservation by not bringing pamphlets and diagrams related to puberty to the parents meeting. This was done to respect their religious beliefs and privacy and because English literacy skills may have been limited. I explained to the parents that the students would be shown posters with drawings of the reproductive system and that the pamphlets which could be used contained drawings and explanations for both males and females. However, the parents were informed that they would first have the opportunity to preview the pamphlets for their acceptance or rejection and distribution would not take place unless their approval was given.

Terms such as "peer pressure" and "teenage rebellion" were not used because these terms would have had little meaning for parents raised in Mexico. For example, I preserved and maintained the parents' traditional values of education and child-rearing which focus on the gradual transition to adult responsibilities. During classes held with the students, discussion was facilitated which supported respect for themselves, their families, and their traditions.

II.   Cultural care accommodation or negotiation "refers to those assistive, supporting, facilitative, or enabling creative professional actions and decisions that help people of a designated culture to adapt to, or to negotiate with, others for a beneficial or satisfying health outcome with professional careproviders" (Leininger, 1991, p. 48). This is a joint process where the clients and the nurse collaborate to arrive at mutually agreed upon actions or decisions. Nurses need to be cognizant of the differences that may exist in the value systems, world views, and definitions of health.

For this mode, I drew upon the culture care meanings of reciprocity, connectedness, and spiritual relatedness. It was important to realize that parents would need to reach a shared decision that was compatible with their religious beliefs. The parents meeting at the Old Colony school involved much negotiation. Classes for both males and females from ages 11–18 were offered and possible topics were briefly described. One parent asked how I would respond if a student inquired about birth control. Recognizing the importance of the parents' respect for religious teachings prohibiting birth control, I replied that the intent was not to provide a "how to" class and that I would respect the parents' decision that birth control methods would not be discussed. After consultation among themselves, the parents requested that classes be taught to the girls fourteen years and older. It was agreed that the female teacher would attend. The parents also requested content on puberty, pregnancy, sexually transmitted diseases and AIDS. They wanted their older daughters to have an understanding of the female reproductive system and an awareness of some of the risks of sexual activity. Concern for the younger girls "finding out too much" was expressed and I was asked to tell the students in the classes not to share the content.

III. Cultural care repatterning or restructuring "refers to those assistive, supporting, facilitative, or enabling professional actions and decisions that help a client(s) reorder, change, or greatly modify their lifeways for new, different, and beneficial health care patterns while respecting the client(s) cultural values and beliefs and still providing a beneficial or healthier lifeway than before the changes were coestablished with the client(s)" (Leininger, 1991, p. 49).

With the third transcultural nursing mode, I utilized the culture care concepts of (1) responsibility and, (2) respect for traditional values, and (3) privacy. The decision to hold the classes rested with the parents; teaching was offered, not imposed. Considering the educational history and the traditional values of privacy and isolation from the world, it was truly an act of repatterning when teaching was requested. Yet the request was consistent with the care value of being responsible for children. Parents expressed their concerns related to their daughters' lack of knowledge and the potential risks of unplanned pregnancies and sexually transmitted diseases. Cultural care repatterning was supported by placing the process of decision making in the context of Old Colony Mennonite care meanings. Because of the value placed on sexual privacy, it would have been unrealistic to assume that all of the classes offered (i.e., to the younger children) would have been initially accepted. Future classes may be requested from the base which has been established.

As a nurse, my professional assumption was that teaching related to puberty and the implications of sexual activity was valuable. However, as a transcultural nurse, I had to be able to work with the culture values and care modalities of the people. I would have had great difficulty had I functioned as a public health nurse without transcultural knowledge and skills. One could have predicted resistance to the proposed classes. Moreover, the goal of culture care would not have been met. As predicted by the Culture Care theory, by working with Old Colony Mennonite parents, teachers and students in culturally appropriate ways, nursing actions directed toward improving health and well being were successfully implemented. It was a sensitive and difficult area for a professional nurse, but my knowledge of transcultural nursing and the use of the Culture Care theory made this experience rewarding and effective with the people.

CONCLUSION

Information was presented to Old Colony Mennonite parents and students in a culturally appropriate way which supported and maintained important care meanings such as *spiritual relatedness*, *respect*, and *presence*, discovered through the theory of Culture Care and use of the ethnonursing research method. As predicted by Leininger's theory of Culture Care Diversity and Universality, nursing care decisions and actions in three modes were generated for specific culture care practices. Based on the care meanings of *reciprocity*, *connectedness*, and *spiritual relatedness*, an acceptable teaching format for all involved was negotiated between the clients and the nurse. Repatterning was facilitated by respecting traditional values, especially being responsible for children and privacy, and involving the parents as coparticipants. All three modes of nursing actions required prior planning, awareness, and thoughtful consideration of the Old Colony Mennonite culture, traditions, and care patterns.

Above all, transcultural nurses must understand the culture in depth when planning and implementing care with clients. As a transcultural nurse, one must be very creative, sensitive and flexible, and draw upon transcultural principles and research findings. The importance of having an understanding of the culture with which one is working, and using a theoretical base cannot be overestimated. It was a rewarding experience as a transcultural nurse to use the Culture Care theory within a public health nursing practice in a school context working with parents, teachers, and students. The Old Colony Mennonite people expressed satisfaction with the benefits of having a transcultural nurse working with them. Only through transcultural knowledge and practices can one insure culture congruent care that leads to the health and well being of clients. This was the goal of the theory of Culture Care and it was substantiated with the Old Colony Mennonites in a number of specific ways.

REFERENCES

Driedger, L. (1986). Mennonite community change: From ethnic en-claves to social networks. *The Mennonite Quarterly Review*, 60(3), 374–386.

Driedger, L. (1988). *Mennonite identity in conflict*. Lewiston and Queen-ston: The Edwin Mellen Press.

Driedger, N. N. (1972). *The Leamington Mennonite Church: Establish-ment and development 1925–1972*. Altona, Canada: D. W. Friesen and Sons.

Dueck, M. (1989). *Mennonite health promotion project*. Grant applica-tion to the Ontario Ministry of Health, Health Promotion Grants Program.

Epp, F. H. (1974). *Mennonites in Canada 1786–1920: The history of a separate people*. Toronto: Macmillan of Canada.

Epp, F. H. (1982). *Mennonites in Canada, 1920–1940: A people's strug-gle for survival*. Toronto: Macmillan of Canada.

Friesen, V. C. (1988). *The windmill turning: Nursery rhymes, maxims, and other expressions of Western Canadian Mennonites*. Edmonton, Canada: The University of Alberta Press.

Horst, J. L. (Ed.) (1934). *Instruction to beginners in the Christian life*. Kitchener, Canada: Herald Press.

Leininger, M. M. (1985a). Transcultural care diversity and univer-sality: A theory of nursing. *Nursing & Health Care*, 6(4), 209–212.

Leininger, M. M. (Ed.) (1985b). *Qualitative research methods in nursing.* Orlando, FL: Grune & Stratton.

Leininger, M. M. (1988). Leininger's theory of nursing: Cultural care diversity and universality. *Nursing Science Quarterly, 1*(4), 152–160.

Leininger, M. M. (Ed.) (1991). *Culture care diversity and universality: A theory of nursing.* New York: National League for Nursing Press.

Redekop, C. W. (1969). *The Old Colony Mennonites: Dilemmas of ethnic minority life.* Baltimore: Johns Hopkins Press.

Sawatzky, H. L (1971). *They sought a country: Mennonite colonization in Mexico.* Berkeley: University of California Press.

Warkentin, A. (1987). *Gaste und fremdlinge: Strangers and pilgrims.* Steinbach, Canada: Die Mennonitische Post/Derksen Printers.

Wenger, A. F., and Wenger, M. (1988). Community and family care patterns of the Old Order Amish. In M. M. Leininger (Ed.), *Care: Discovery and uses in clinical and community nursing* (pp. 39–54). Detroit: Wayne State University Press.

11

Nursing Guatemalan Families
Using Leininger's Culture Care Theory

Charlotte D. Barry
Patricia B. Kronk

Madeleine Leininger's theory of Cultural Diversity and Universality provided the caring philosophy for this ethnonursing project, which unfolded into a rich mosaic of human caring. The focus of transcultural nursing is the study of people from different cultures in the world with thought to the ways the nurse can assist people with their daily health and living needs (Leininger, 1978). Discovery of nursing knowledge focused on cultural care, preservation, accommodation and repatterning emerges from the client's world view, and from knowing the other as person and client, and knowing self as person and nurse.

PURPOSE OF THE STUDY

The purpose of this mini ethnographic study was to gain knowledge of the Guatemalan culture, health care beliefs, concept of health and caring behaviors, and their barriers to health care. The specific purpose of the study was to create a cultural model of care for the Guatemalan

The authors wish to express their gratitude to Lois Kelley, PhD, RN, Assistant Professor, Florida Atlantic University College of Nursing, for guiding their journey to Citrustown, and to Marilyn Ray, PhD, RN, Associate Professor and Eminent Scholar in Nursing, Florida Atlantic University College of Nursing, for assisting in the final preparation of this manuscript.

families in Citrustown, a fictitious name for a city in the Southeastern United States.

HISTORICAL OVERVIEW OF THE GUATEMALAN PEOPLE

In 1982 a group of Guatemalan refugees, descendants of ancient Mayan Indians, began arriving in Citrustown (Ashabranner, 1986). They sought refuge from political unrest, persecution and extreme poverty in Guatemala (Menchú, 1984). Bermudez (1986) describes the Guatemalan government's systematic relocation of the Mayan Indians to "model communities" further into the forest and highlands, where farming would be next to impossible. Many of these refugees walked across Mexico and hitchhiked across the United States to Citrustown. Others were brought by "coyotes," men, who for a fee, transport Central Americans to safe havens in the United States (Ashabranner, 1986). Subsistence farmers in Guatemala, these Mayan refugees have become farm laborers in Citrustown, a sleepy, one stoplight town surrounded by 50,000 fertile acres of citrus groves, vegetable fields, and grazing land. Employment is mainly agricultural, with the two East Coast migrant streams beginning and ending here. The migrant streams follow the sun and travel as far north as central New York and Michigan (Smith & Gentry, 1987). This migratory lifeway mirrors the Mayans' migration to coffee and cotton plantations on the Guatemalan coast (Menchú, 1984).

The Mayan Indians speak twenty-four dialects in Guatemala (Ashabranner, 1986). Kanjobal is the dialect spoken by the Mayans in Citrustown. The division of the Mayan group by language in Guatemala lends itself to factionalism, preventing a unified front to fight oppression (Ashabranner, 1986). This indigenous Indian dialect isolates these Mayan refugees within the Citrustown community.

DOMAIN OF INQUIRY

Nurses in the primary health center located in this rural community identified communication as a major barrier to providing nursing care to the Guatemalans. Although several of the personnel at the primary health center spoke fluent or "get-by" Spanish, no one spoke or understood Kanjobal. The lifeways of this culture group remained unknown.

The nurses related stories of improper use of medications by this culture group. Because of the language barrier, instructions were sketchy and probably not fully understood. The pharmacy in town dispensed the prescriptions in English, with English instructions. Women were known to have poured liquid antibiotics into babies' ears for ear infections and antibiotic capsules were opened and the contents spread on the skin of an infected foot.

A trilingual worker at the church-supported social service center confirmed that there was much confusion among the Guatemalans about medications as they would often stop there after clinic visits for clarification of instructions. The principal of the elementary school validated confusion regarding medications and reported that children known to be taking medications rarely brought the medication to school for daytime dosages.

The nurses in the county public health clinic supported the notion that language was a major barrier to health care and understanding the lifeways of the Mayan refugees, which contributed to the isolation of the Guatemalan population in Citrustown. One incident observed by the researchers involved a young Guatemalan mother who had contracted gonorrhea. She and her 11 day old infant had received an injection of Rocephan at the health center two days before, and had not yet filled their prescriptions for Erythromycin. She said she was unable to walk to the pharmacy. Another incident occurred during a home visit, and involved a liquid antibiotic. The medication instructions read "refrigerate after opening," but the bottle was sitting out on a table in the living room and was warm to the touch.

The researchers gained personal insight into the isolation experienced by these refugees during a home visit with the social worker from the county public health department, further corroborating the notion of language as a barrier to professional health care. Magdalena's story is a poignant accounting of a life experience, and illustrates the patterns of needs, expressions of values, and human responses (Leininger, 1985).

Magdalena's Story

Number 27, Sandy Camp, was the home of Magdalena C., a 21 year-old female refugee from political oppression and poverty in Guatemala. Nine months pregnant, with no prenatal care, she arrived in Citrustown with her husband and 16-month-old daughter. They moved in with her mother-in-law who was blind since birth, her sister and brother-in-law and their two children, and another brother and sister-in-law and their two children. Magdalena's husband went to work in the fields. Their home was a three bedroom, sparsely furnished unit with electricity, indoor plumbing, and cold running water. There was a telephone in the house. The family all spoke Kanjobal. The men also spoke some Spanish.

Magdalena felt the baby move on Sunday. The following Wednesday, at 4:00 P.M., she delivered a still-born baby boy at home. Her husband was working in the fields, her mother-in-law was home but was unable to use the telephone to call for help. Magdalena wrapped the baby in a blanket and held him until her husband came home from work at 7:00 P.M. He then called for help. The ambulance arrived and took the mother and infant to the County Hospital. The mother was released later that night, but the infant's body was kept at the hospital.

The social worker visited Magdalena the following day. She spoke no Kanjobal, but was, however, fluent in Spanish and was able to communicate with Magdalena through her husband. The new mother huddled on her bed, wrapped in a blanket, was pale and drained of energy. She cried when she asked for help to find her baby's body.

The researchers were challenged to explore the Guatemalan culture, health beliefs, and caring practices of these persons in order to create a model for nursing the Guatemalan families in Citrustown.

LITERATURE REVIEW

The literature search included articles on Guatemalan refugees, Guatemalan culture, migrant health problems, health care in developing countries, and medication compliance. Kita (1988), a Maryknoll missionary who lived among the people in the highlands of Guatemala, described their lifeways. In a telephone interview in 1988, Kita detailed their health care beliefs. They included seeking the advice of native curers, preference for herbal medications and pomades, and a mystical belief in the power of injections. She also related that the Mayan refugees would have a difficult time adhering to a medication schedule expressed as hours in the day because in Guatemala, they generally do not have clocks and tell time by the phases of the sun and moon. Early's monograph (1982) adds further insight into the Guatemalan culture and health care beliefs. He stated in an interview (1988) that Western medical practices have been adopted in Guatemala and these professional health services are utilized in conjunction with shamans and traditional healing beliefs. He confirmed Kita's view about injections and further stated that Guatemalans would be reluctant to take oral medications or, conversely, might take the entire prescription at one time. Lewis (1966) in his seminal work about the "culture of poverty" described time orientation centered in the present and the past, with very little thought given to the future.

Smith and Gentry (1987) identified farm workers as having the poorest health of any group in the United States. Higher rates of respiratory infections, tuberculosis, parasites and occupational health problems are further aggravated by a lifestyle that involves difficult physical labor, low wages, exposure to the weather, substandard living quarters and constant need to move from place to place. Social isolation results from cultural differences, language barriers and inadequate education and translates into anxiety, depression and a feeling of hopelessness (Smith & Gentry, 1987). Loneliness and social isolation are experienced by immigrant women and are not relieved over time, as feelings of marginality, not really belonging to either their homeland or their new country, contribute to depression (Anderson, 1985).

Mirales (1986) studied the Guatemalan population in Southeast United States and described health care beliefs that focused on conditions of hot or cold as the cause of illness. When illness occurred, the Guatemalan refugees first used over the counter drugs, then consulted with native curers, and finally sought help from the professional system in the community. Boyle (1985) studied health care beliefs and illness behaviors of 22 households in the central highlands of western Guatemala and determined that the individual's psychological state or extreme emotional state involving anger, sadness, grief, passion or fright could contribute to illness. Conditions of hot or cold have traditionally been viewed by Spanish culture groups as external forces of nature that cause illness. This was confirmed in her research (Boyle, 1985).

Medication compliance is affected by cultural beliefs about health, disease and effectiveness of medication (Pecori, 1987). Socio-economic factors, income, transportation and age, can influence compliance. Patient education involving the nature of the illness, action of the medication, and information on how and when to take the medications can have a positive effect on medication compliance (Pecori, 1987).

Werner (1977) provided an explicit text of common health care problems and treatments as a guide for village health care workers in developing countries. Using phases of the moon and sun, Werner (1977) developed a medication information tool and presented it as a means for understanding medication administration schedules. This medication tool offered by Werner to be used by the readers seemed to be an appropriate educational tool for the Guatemalan refugees in Citrustown.

SETTING AND SAMPLE

A primary health care center in this rural community provided the setting for this study. During the four months that the researchers were engaged in the study, information was gathered from several sources. Key informants were the nurses at the primary health care center, and the nurses and a social worker at the county public health clinic. Workers at the social service center, the principal of the elementary school, and a Catholic priest also informed the researchers. Four Guatemalan women participated in a health beliefs inquiry and evaluation of Werner's (1977) medication information tool. The informants were obtained in a serendipitous manner. Lack of telephones, the unpredictable opportunity of field work, and the availability of an interpreter, precluded the firm scheduling of appointments. All of the women spoke Kanjobal, and one woman also spoke English and Spanish. Three of the women were married, one was not, and all lived in multi-family dwellings.

Three interviews were conducted in the informants' homes, using two different interpreters. One informant also spoke English, and that interview was conducted at the social service center.

METHODOLOGY

Leininger defines ethnonursing as a specific nursing research method and offers the "Sunrise Model" as a framework for knowledge generation (Leininger, 1978). (See "Sunrise Model" in Chapter Nine.) Data generation methods of observation, interview, life history, photography and participation with the people in their own environment, assisted the researchers to enter the world of the other in order to bridge the gap between the folk health system and the professional health system.

The Research Process

The researchers prepared to enter the world of the other by assuming a deliberate and active learning role. "Learning about, listening to, and observing are the dominant roles of the ethnonursing researcher (Leininger, 1985, p. 53)." The four phases of ethnonursing research are observation, participation, interviewing and validating data (Leininger, 1985).

The researchers drove to the community and casually observed the town and its inhabitants. Like sightseers, the schools, housing, shops, churches, parks, ball fields, industry and tourist attractions were explored. Observations were documented in field notes and maintained in a journal. The notes recorded observations, direct quotes, time spent in the field, content of phone conversations, interviews, and the context and details of participation.

The primary work of the observation phase is inquiry and listening. Several interviews were conducted, both casual and deliberate, with health care workers familiar with the Guatemalans in Citrustown. Other interviews were conducted with social workers, teachers, nuns, priests, an anthropologist, a housing inspector, community workers, and cooperative founder. The interview process proved to be a critical pathway to knowing the Guatemalans as each informant recommended another informant or resource, i.e., book, newspaper article, journal or thesis. A photo journal, reflecting the living environments, family communications and other lifeways of the people, was also used to study this culture group.

Participant observation was restricted by the length of the project, however, the researchers did attend the annual harvest festival, a Kanjobal Mass, made home visits with the social worker, and worked side by side with nurses in the clinics.

Semi-structured interviews were conducted with four Guatemalan women. The questionnaire was designed to elicit information about health care beliefs, caring practices and evaluation of Werner's (1977) Medication Information Tool. Examples of the questions include: What does health mean to you? What do you do for your family to make them feel better? What do the nurses do to make you feel better? Do you see your children's lives as being better than yours?

The interviews were conducted with the assistance of interpreters who were invaluable in helping the researchers and participants bridge the communication barrier. The interpreters facilitated the responses of the participants and clarified the meanings of the responses for the researchers. An ongoing process of validation was employed as findings were discussed with key informants or compared to findings in the literature. Validity in qualitative research refers to gaining knowledge and understanding of the phenomenon under investigation and preserving the "heart and flesh of the data" (Leininger, 1985, p.69).

The three hour round trip car ride to Citrustown afforded the researchers time to reflect on observations, discuss current journal readings, and review the plans for the day. At the end of the day the ninety minute car ride home again gave the reseachers an opportunity to reflect on the day's work, add observations to the field notes, and consider the next phase of the study.

DATA ANALYSIS

Content analysis was used to analyze the data. The data were studied for characteristics and divided into categories according to the framework of the "Sunrise Model." The researchers attempted to accurately describe the data within these categories in order to present a portrayal of the lifeways of the Guatemalan refugees in Citrustown. The results of the Health Beliefs Interviews are described within the context of the informants' responses and by the themes that emerged from the data. The understanding of the Medication Information Tool (Figure 11.1) is also described within the context of the informants' responses. The photo journal was edited for repetition and clarity of the images.

GENERAL FINDINGS

The Guatemalans in Citrustown have come to the United States with a broad range of beliefs, values, and ideas. Health and illness are part of their culture and must be approached and appreciated from a holistic and humanistic view. "Understanding how social structure, world view, environment, and folk and professional health care systems influence nursing is essential to obtain a holistic picture of the people and their actual or potential nursing needs" (Leininger, 1985, p.58).

Dosage Blank
For giving medicine to those people who cannot read

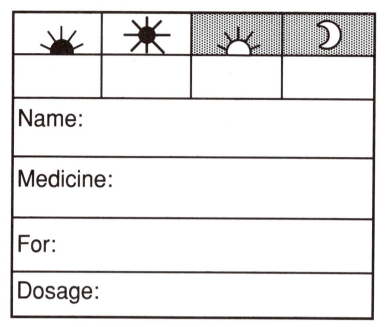

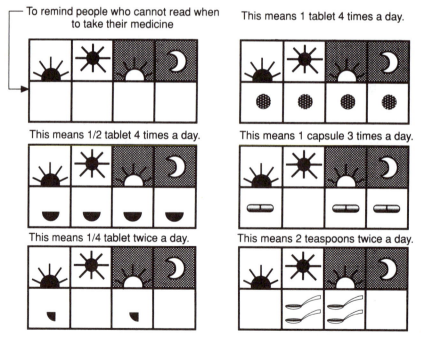

To remind people who cannot read when to take their medicine

This means 1 tablet 4 times a day.

This means 1/2 tablet 4 times a day.

This means 1 capsule 3 times a day.

This means 1/4 tablet twice a day.

This means 2 teaspoons twice a day.

Note: From *Where There is No Doctor: A Village Health Care Handbook* (p. 63) by D. Werner, 1977. Palo Alto, CA: Hesperian Foundation. Copyright 1977 by The Hesperian Foundation. Adapted by permission.

Figure 11.1 Medication Information Tool.

Social Structure Aspects

Kinship/Social Factors   The Mayan Indians are easily recognized in Citrustown by their short stature and distinctive dress. The men wear long sleeved shirts, jeans and baseball caps, and can often be seen walking in twos or threes along the highway, carrying small white plastic grocery bags. The women are usually dressed in long, colorful skirts, and short sleeved cotton tops. On holidays and festivals they wear traditional garb: long, vibrant colored, handwoven wraparound skirts called "cortes" and hand-embroidered blouses called "huipils." The women have long, black, shiny hair which, according to tradition cannot be cut. The Guatemalan community is very young, with an average age being 18.8 years and the average family having 2.3 children (Mirales, 1986). Young mothers were frequently seen walking through town carrying their babies papoose-style in hand-woven blankets. These people appeared solemn and shy. Many women marry by the age of 14 and give birth to their first child at the age of 15 (Mirales, 1986).

Social activities revolve around the Catholic Church, with a men's soccer team and the annual Festival de San Miguel. This festival, the main social event of the year, is held every October on the church grounds. It is a traditional celebration of the harvest, with a parade, crowning of queens, music, food and the selling of wares. Women seem to have no social life outside the structure of the family.

The majority of Guatemalans live in multiple family rental units called Sandy Camp, Sea Camp, and Shell Camp. Each unit houses two to three different families who share common kitchen and bathroom facilities. Privacy is maintained by use of hanging curtains, sheets or other types of screening as partitions.

The camps come under the "boarding house" category described by the Housing Authority, and therefore allow the landlord to charge rent per head, per week. Single men usually live in rooms with several other men. Shell Camp has running water, hot plates for cooking, and no heat. Sandy Camp has no hot water and no heat. Sea Camp, also known as "Roach Palace," has no heat, falling-down ceilings and walls, and a generally unsafe appearance. Some Guatemalans have moved into single homes and trailers, but always with one or more other families. The Housing Inspector responds to complaints of unsafe housing. However, he states that given the quiet, shy nature of the Guatemalans and the shortage of housing in Citrustown, few complaints are filed and unsafe and unsanitary conditions persist.

Economic Factors   Life in Citrustown is of a subsistence system. Most men work as farm laborers, earning low wages, and many of the women also work in the fields. Depending on the season, tomatoes, peppers or flowers are picked. Agricultural workers are exempt from minimum wage laws. Their days are long and the work is hard. The day begins at sun-up and does not end until sun-down. Meals are often carried into the fields, consisting of traditional food such as tortillas, supplemented with soup and cold drinks, such as water or Coca Cola. The women who remain at home often mind the children of those who work in the fields for a fee of $5.00 per day.

A clothing cooperative has been formed to provide year-round work in town, thereby allowing one member of the family to stay at home year round. It is thought that this would keep the children in school and help break the migrant cycle. The co-op imports Guatemalan fabrics and makes native clothing to be sold at local shops and in catalogues. The workers also do contract work making clothing for wholesalers. The co-op employs about 20 people, with hopes to expand.

Educational Factors   Elementary school and middle school education is provided by the county school system. A Migrant Head Start Day Care program from birth to kindergarten is federally funded. It is open from November to May to meet the needs of the migrating farm workers. New Hope Rural School, grades one through four, is funded by donations, housed at the Holy Cross Catholic Church grounds, and provides education to migrant and non-migrant children.

Although it is usually open from November through May, recently it has remained open the entire school year to accommodate those children who stay in town and do not migrate. English classes are held at the Catholic Church in the evening during the week, and many women have learned to write their names at classes held at the different "camps."

Political Factors   The social service center acts as an information and referral agency which helps new arrivals to adjust to life in Citrustown. One of its main functions is the processing of immigration applications, but the workers at the center also teach the newly arriving immigrants to use the laundromat, post office, supermarket, indoor plumbing and endless other activities of daily living.

Religious Factors   There are several churches in Citrustown, however the majority of Guatemalans are Catholic. A Kanjobal Mass is said every Saturday and a Spanish Mass is said on Sunday. Native music is played at the Mass on an ancient Mayan musical instrument called a marimba.

Cultural Values and Belief Factors   Beliefs are embedded in ancient Mayan traditions which foster family life, care of the children, respect for elders and a strong sense of self-respect. Disgrace is brought on the family by publicly breaking an observed tradition.

Folk/Traditional Health Care Factors   Folk practices by native curers remain, for the most part, clandestine, but seem to consist of compounds and potions made from native Guatemalan herbs.

Professional Health Care Factors   The Community Health Center is a funded primary health care center for the indigent. Fees are on a sliding scale, and prescriptions are often paid for by the clinic. The primary health center provides dental and medical care and laboratory services. According to health care records, the most common illnesses experienced by the Guatemalan refugees are upper respiratory infections, skin diseases, parasites, tuberculosis, pesticide poisoning, sexually transmitted diseases, and occupational accidents.

The public health clinic provides pre-natal care, a well-baby clinic, immunizations, family planning, school nursing and immigration physicals. The WIC (Women, Infants and Children) program provides nutritional help to the community through education and vouchers for cereal, milk, cheese, formula and juice. Eligibility for this program is for pregnant women and children up to the age of five. The IPO (Improved Pregnancy Outcome) is another educational program sponsored at the clinic. Hospitalizations and childbirth take place at the county hospital.

ETHNOHEALTH FINDINGS

All the informants had difficulty answering the questions, with the exception of the demographic section. Health was defined by two informants as when they were "happy." One woman described health as when she was able to care for her babies. One woman was unable to define health.

The five most frequently described illnesses were fever, coughing, headaches, diarrhea, and back pains. Back pain was associated with childbirth and farm work. Diarrhea was associated with eating American food. The one English speaking informant described headaches as being associated with depression caused by feelings of isolation, separation from family, boredom or receiving bad news from home. At the time of illness all the informants stated they would try home remedies first, i.e., cold showers, orange juice, and over-the-counter drugs. They would then seek the advice of a native curer. Advice from the Professional Health system would be sought last.

All the informants stated that the doctors cared for them by giving them prescriptions, and the nurses cared for them by giving them treatments. The informants described caring for others in time of illness by preparing food for them, and further described their own feelings of being cared for when others in turn prepared food. All the informants viewed their own lives as being better in ten years and predicted their children's lives will be better through education. They all believed their children will not work in the fields. Themes emerged that could provide direction for further nursing research, and include caring through food, hope for a better life for their children through education, isolation and somatization and the role of women in this culture.

Each informant expressed understanding of the Medication Information Tool and the symbolic expressions of time. The nurses at the health center and the workers at the service center all understood the Medication Information Tool and viewed it as an educational tool that would facilitate patients' understanding of medications and treatment schedules.

PRESENTATION OF FINDINGS TO HEALTH CARE PERSONNEL

The findings of this study were presented to the nursing staff at the primary health center. A slide presentation of the photo journal afforded the staff an opportunity to experience the living conditions of the Guatemalan refugees in Citrustown, and begin the discovery of knowing these people. The researchers provided the staff with descriptions of the Guatemalan culture, health care beliefs and values, and encouraged the staff to reflect on the possibilities of nursing across cultural barriers. The Medication Information Tool was explained to the staff and blank copies were presented to them for their use. A felt board depicting the medication tool was constructed by the researchers and presented to the nursing staff as a visual aid for teaching the Guatemalan refugees about their medication and treatment schedules.

RECOMMENDATIONS OF THE STUDY

Culture sensitive nursing care, respectful and supportive of existing health care practices and beliefs, would reduce barriers to health care for the Guatemalan refugees in Citrustown. Some knowledge of the language would facilitate nursing care at the health centers. A lay community health worker would strengthen an outreach program for follow-up care for those unable to come to the center. Participation of members of the community, including folk curers, in collaboration with the professional health system, would facilitate provision of health care services designed to meet the health needs of the community as they are described by the community. Health promotion requires nurses to become involved in issues affecting the environment and empowering others to become responsible for their own health. Transcultural nursing challenges nurses to consider such issues as poverty, nutrition, education, housing, transportation, and justice as they nurse persons from different cultures and assist them with their daily health and living needs.

REFERENCES

Anderson, J. M. (1985). Perspectives on the health of immigrant women: A feminist analysis. *Advances in Nursing Science, 8*(1), 61–76.

Ashabranner, B. (1986). *Children of the Maya: A Guatemalan Indian Odyssey.* New York: Dodd, Mead & Company.

Bermudez, F. (1986). *Life and death in Guatemala.* New York: Orvis Press.

Boyle, J. (1985). Use of the family health calendar and interview schedules to study health and illness. In M. Leininger (Ed.), *Qualitative research methods in nursing* (pp. 217–235). New York: Grune & Stratton, Inc.

Early, J. (1982). Some structures of demographic transition (Mortality). *State of Florida Board of Regents*, pp. 96–130.

Kita, B. (1988). *What prize awaits us.* New York: Orvis Press.

Leininger, M. (1978). *Transcultural nursing: Concepts, theories and practices.* New York: John Wiley & Sons.

Leininger, M. (1985). Ethnography and ethnonursing: Models and modes of qualitative data analysis. In M. Leininger (Ed.), *Qualitative research methods in nursing* (pp. 33–71). New York: Grune & Stratton, Inc.

Lewis, O. (1966). *La Vida: A Puerto Rican family in the culture of poverty in San Juan and New York.* New York: Random House.

Menchú, R. (1984). *I, Rigoberta Menchú—An Indian woman in Guatemala.* E. Burgos-Debray (Ed.). New York: Verso Books.

Mirales, M. (1986). *Health seeking behavior of Guatemalan refugees in South Florida* (Unpublished Master's Thesis). Gainesville, FL: University of Florida.

Pecori, P. (1987). *The relationship of health beliefs of patients with hypertension to their compliance with a prescribed medication regime* (Unpublished Master's Thesis). Pittsburgh, PA: University of Pittsburgh.

Smith, L., & Gentry, D. (1987). Migrant farm workers' perceptions of support persons in a descriptive community survey. *Public Health Nursing, 4*(1), 21–28.

Werner, D. (1977). *Where there is no doctor: A Village health care handbook.* Palo Alto, CA: Hesperian Foundation.

Part VI

Watson's Theory of Transpersonal Caring

12

Cost Effectiveness of a Theory-Based Nurse-Managed Center for Persons Living with HIV/AIDS

Carole Schroeder

The purpose of this chapter is to explore cost effectiveness of the Denver Nursing Project in Human Caring, a nurse-managed outpatient center for persons living with Human Immune Deficiency Virus (HIV) and Acquired Immune Deficiency Syndrome (AIDS). Also called the Caring Center, the Denver Nursing Project is based on Jean Watson's theory of nursing as the art and science of human caring (1985a, 1985b, 1988, 1990). Watson views caring as a moral ideal in nursing, and believes that human beings possess inner resources and strengths that can be called upon to meet health challenges. Care is primary to cure in Watson's theory, and the work has particular relevance for nurses caring for persons living with HIV/AIDS.

The nurses at the Caring Center are concerned with helping clients maintain a supportable quality of life during the disease of HIV/AIDS; relationship is considered primary at the Center. The majority of services offered at the Caring Center are independent nursing services such as teaching, assessment and referral, coordination of services, and consultation aimed at preventing hospital admissions, and decreasing prolonged inpatient hospital stays. Less than 25 percent of services offered at the Center are traditional medically supportive services such as administration of blood transfusions, and IV fluids and medications. Thus, it is inappropriate to compare the Caring Center with outpatient infectious disease clinics providing only medically supportive treatments.

Because of the uniqueness of the Center, a variety of methods were used to determine the impact of the Center on health care costs. Initially, the current status of nurse-managed centers in the United States will be outlined, as will the operations and funding structure of the Center. Problems inherent in determining cost effectiveness of the Center will then be discussed. Next, the incidence and costs of HIV/ AIDS in the U.S. and Colorado will be presented; these numbers will be used to estimate public health cost savings that are a result of the Center's nursing services. The cost saving estimates will be supported by presenting results of quantitative and qualitative evaluation research projects conducted at the Center.

ABOUT NURSE-MANAGED CENTERS

Nurse-managed centers are unique in that clients have direct access to nursing services without having to pay a physician referral fee. Nurse-managed centers provide a wide range of outpatient care services, and usually emphasize assessment and screening, education and counseling, consultation, and maintenance of home care. The National League for Nursing (NLN) defines a nurse-managed center as one in which

> "the nurse occupies . . . a chief management position in the center. . . . Accountability and responsibility for client care and professional practice remain with the nurse. . . . The client has direct access to nursing services."
>
> (Community Nursing Centers, 1992, p. 70).

The number of nurse-managed centers is rapidly increasing in the United States, and currently, about 250 such centers in the United States provide health care to Americans. Over half of these centers are less than five years old ("Community Nursing Center," 1992). In an NLN survey, it was found that nursing care is paid in a variety of ways: 19 percent of charges paid by private insurance, 25 percent paid privately, 24 percent paid by Medicaid or Medicare, 13 percent unreimbursed, and 17 percent reimbursed by other methods. Cost of the average visit is $78.00. Unlike hospitals, there are no shortages of nurses to staff these centers, and these nurses are better paid and better educated than registered nurses nationwide. Due to their focus on prevention, nurse-managed centers have been demonstrated to reduce the cost of care. The National League for Nursing recently stated that nursing centers are "filling a critical void in the nation's health care system" (*Nurse-Run Centers*, 1992, p. 70).

ABOUT THE DENVER NURSING PROJECT IN HUMAN CARING

The idea for the Denver Nursing Project in Human Caring was conceived by hospital nurses concerned that the needs of this vulnerable population were not being met in acute care settings. The Center uses Jean Watson's work on nursing and caring as the basis for education, clinical practice and research; it is utilized 450-550 times per month, primarily by homosexual men living with HIV/AIDS. Since 1988, the Center has recorded more than 14,000 outpatient visits, and the number of visits increases monthly. The majority of the Center's clients' HIV/AIDS health care costs are paid by public programs such as the Veterans' Administration, Medicaid, or Colorado State Aid to the Medically Indigent.

Nursing services are comprehensive at the Center, and comprise both independent and medically supportive nursing services. Independent nursing services include therapeutic touch, massage, counseling, nursing care partnerships (a form of nursing case management), and individual and group education regarding all aspects of living with HIV/AIDS. Medically supportive services include fluid, blood, and medication administration, laboratory work, and wound care. Client support groups are ongoing at the Center, and most nursing services include clients and their lovers, families and friends. In addition, the Center participates as a clinical placement site for nursing, medical and dental students.

Funding of the Center

Three local hospitals and the University of Colorado School of Nursing Center for Human Caring initiated financial support for the Center. Persons eligible to participate in the services at the Center receive their HIV/AIDS primary care through one of three hospitals which sponsor the Center. At first, one hospital provided the majority of clients and financial support to the Center, donating a building, office supplies and support services, and a part-time infection control nurse. Then, two other local hospitals augmented the Center, each providing a part-time clinical nurse. The University of Colorado School of Nursing, Center for Human Caring provided consultation in nursing theory, grant writing, and limited financial support.

In 1990, the Department of Health and Human Services, Division of Nursing, awarded substantial federal grant funding to the Center. This support was awarded in order to increase client access to nursing services and to investigate the viability of a nurse-managed center for persons with HIV/AIDS. It also allowed expansion of the scope of services offered at the Center, including the hiring of a clinical director, registered nurses, clinical nurse specialists, a secretary, administrative coordinator, and a research coordinator. After four years of operation, numerous evaluation research projects and testimonials, the Center has been determined to be an important and well-utilized option in health care delivery for persons living with HIV/AIDS (Schroeder & Maeve, 1992; Schroeder & Neil, 1992; Neil & Schroeder, 1992). However, the financial viability and cost effectiveness of the Center has not yet been determined. Accordingly, as the Center nears the last year of its three-year funding period, determination of cost effectiveness has become a priority.

THE PROBLEM OF DETERMINING COST EFFECTIVENESS OF A NURSE-MANAGED CENTER

The Center is unique in many aspects: in its caring theory-based, nurse-managed model of HIV/AIDS practice; in its dual funding model which is based on the consortium and a federal grant; unlike other nursing centers, the Center does not employ nurse practitioners, instead utilizing doctoral, masters, or baccalaureate prepared registered nurses in its professional practice. Moreover, unlike most outpatient HIV/AIDS centers, the majority of services offered are not traditional physician-ordered medical treatments. Less than 25 percent of the services offered at the Center are reimbursable, medically supportive services (requiring a physician's order) such as laboratory work, intravenous fluid replacement, blood transfusions, etc. Over 75 percent of the Center's nursing services are independent services (performed by nurses independent of physicians), aimed at client self care, prevention of complications, and maintenance of a supportable and humane quality of life throughout the course of the disease. In addition, these services assist clients and caregivers to negotiate the health care system as informed and knowledgeable consumers. A major aim of the Center is to provide health-related services and education which enable clients to remain out of hospitals for as long as possible. Although the nursing services are relatively inexpensive and substantially reduce hospital costs, (owing to the elimination of physician involvement) they are not considered reimbursable by federal or state funded health care programs such as Medicaid or Colorado State Aid to the Medically Indigent.

Thus, because of its emphasis on prevention, it is extremely difficult to quantify cost effectiveness of the Center's programs. As a consequence, this exploration of the impact of the Denver Nursing Project on HIV/AIDS health care costs will use a variety of quantitative and qualitative means to estimate costs saving.

INCIDENCE AND COSTS OF HIV/AIDS IN THE U.S. AND COLORADO

In the United States, more than one million people are estimated to be infected with HIV/AIDS (Barnes, 1992), and over 230,000 cases have been reported to the Center for Disease Control as of June 1992. Colorado ranks 18th among the United States in incidence of HIV/AIDS (Green, 1991), with 2275 cases reported. Colorado hospital charges average $1400 per day for persons hospitalized with HIV/AIDS. Lifetime medical costs of HIV/AIDS are currently estimated to be $102,000 per patient per year (Hellinger, 1992). These figures are presented in Tables 12.1–12.3.

Table 12.1   Total Incidence of HIV/AIDS in US, Colorado and Denver Metropolitan Area Through June 1992

(CDC Monthly AIDS Report/Colorado AIDS Surveillance Report)

	U.S.	Colorado	Denver Metro
Total Cases	230,179	2275	1952

Table 12.2   Costs of HIV/AIDS in US

Total Direct and Indirect Costs*	$66.4 billion
Average Lifetime Medical Costs	$102,000/person
Estimated Costs of *HIV* Care	$10,000/pt/year
Estimated Costs of AIDS InPt. Care	$38,300/yr/pt

("AIDS treatment tab")

*Direct costs include all treatment costs of AIDS, education, research, preventative services, etc.; indirect costs include costs of increased morbidity and mortality on productivity (Green, 1991).

Table 12.3   Incidence & Costs of HIV/AIDS Hospitalizations in Colorado 1991

(Colorado Hospital Association report for June 1991)

	Colorado	Hospitals Which Refer to Caring Center		
		1	2	3
Total number Hospital Admits	1151	346	153	85
% of Colorado Admits*	100%	30%	13%	7%
Average LOS	7.72 days	7.36 days	11.26 days	6.68 days
Av. Charge/Day	$1424	$1229	**	$1822
Total InPt. (Hosp.) Days	9423	2546	1722	568

*The three referring hospitals for the Denver Nursing Project in Human Caring account for 50 percent of Colorado HIV/AIDS hospital admissions and charges.
**Average costs (not charges) for a medical patient day per hospital is $671 (no charges available for HIV/AIDS hospitalization).

QUANTITATIVE SAVINGS OF THE NURSE-MANAGED CENTER

The average daily hospital charge for HIV/AIDS care is $1400; it is indisputable that a program such as the Center (which is able to prevent or decrease prolonged hospital stays) saves enormous amounts of money in public health funds very quickly. Savings in hospital charges for 1991 resulting from the Center's nursing services are estimated at greater than $700,000 in prevented hospital admissions and readmissions, and decreased prolonged hospital stays. This figure was based on the following assumptions:

1. Through the nursing care partnership program of consultation, client and caregiver education, discharge planning and teaching for home care, the Center was estimated to prevent one hospital stay (average charge $10,000) in 20 percent of its patients last year for a savings of approximately $480,000.

2. In 20 percent of its patients, the Center was able to decrease length of stay by one day of one hospitalization for a savings of approximately............................$67,200.

3. Outpatient medical treatments and nursing care partner services performed at the Center prevent hospital inpatient days and readmissions so that one hospital inpatient day saved by each of 50 percent of the 1991 treatments would result in a savings of approximately......................$186,200

Using the foregoing model, an extremely conservative estimate shows potential savings of not less than $733,400.

Supporting Data

Prevention of Hospital Admissions   In this analysis, hospital charges, rather than costs, were used to determine all savings estimates. Forty percent of the total number of clients served were considered to have been hospitalized during a given year. The average number of hospital stays per AIDS patient is 1.8 per year (Green, 1991). Thus, for this analysis, a conservative estimate of 20 percent (48 patients) of the current 240 clients was used to figure cost savings. If the Center were able to prevent one hospital stay for 20 percent of its clients, an average savings of $10,000 per patient/per hospital stay would be realized. A cumulative total savings in charges resulting from the prevention of one admission in 20 percent of the Center's patients in one year equals $480,000.

Decreased Number of Prolonged Hospitalizations   The Center is also able to prevent prolonged hospital stays of its clients, due to the nursing care partnership program which teaches clients and caregivers how to maintain home care and supports their efforts. The nursing care partnership program (NCP) is a third generation form of nursing case management, based on relationship, advocacy, mutuality and empowerment of clients and nurses. The nursing care partnership program saves inpatient hospital costs because nurses provide emotional support through care partnership relationships. They also teach clients and caregivers how to manage symptoms, prevent disease complications, and practice self care. All of these services encourage and nurture home care as an alternative to hospital care. Nursing care partners also visit patients in the hospital to facilitate discharge planning and client wishes with respect to living wills. Many clients carry a wallet sized card from the Center which, when presented upon hospital admission, requests hospital staff to call his or her nursing care partner to consult on care. Because nursing care partners are usually the most informed health professionals regarding the patients' current physical and emotional state, they are at the same time most highly qualified to coordinate the needs expressed through living wills. Thus, prolonged hospitalization periods are avoided.

Clients are frequently discharged early from hospitals to the care of the Center for assessment and to learn home care skills, IV fluid and medication administration, pain management techniques, nutrition, and other skills. The nursing care and nursing care partnership relationships described here have been very successful, as determined by evaluation research projects conducted at the Center. A conservative estimate of savings is one day of one stay (average cost $1400) in 20 percent of the Centers' clients. This is a savings of $67,200.

Cost Savings of Nursing Centers Performing Medically Supportive Treatments   Inpatient hospital treatment is substantially more costly than outpatient treatment for both the general population and for persons living with HIV/AIDS. Outpatient charges are usually one quarter to one half of inpatient charges for similar medical treatments. In 1991, Green determined that the average outpatient charge of $287 for HIV/ AIDS treatment was about one fourth inpatient charges, when compared to the $1400 charge for an average one day stay in a hospital. Fuerst (1991) studied outpatient Pentamidine treatment and fluid replacement of persons with HIV/AIDS, and found that outpatient treatment is substantially less costly than inpatient treatment for the same services. The fact that the Center provides medical treatments in an outpatient setting rather than an inpatient setting assures that costs are being saved for these treatments.

A generous estimate of the Center's operating costs is that they are approximately one half of inpatient medical costs. In 1991, the Center performed 822 medically supportive treatments, 531 of which are complex and usually done in a hospital setting (blood transfusions, IV fluid and medication administration, and Pentamidine treatments). One quarter of these 531 treatments were estimated to result in one saved hospital day per treatment. Based on these figures, a savings of $186,200 is estimated to result from the Center's outpatient medical treatments alone. What is more important, in a recent client survey, 100 percent of respondents preferred to have medical treatments performed at the Center on an outpatient basis, rather than in a hospital. Consequently, by performing medical treatments at the nursing center, patient needs, both emotional and financial, are recognized and responded to, while at the same time, public health care costs are reduced.

Evaluation Research Projects
Regarding Nursing Care Partnerships and Cost Savings

In 1991–1992, two evaluation projects were completed at the Center. In the first, a survey eliciting clients views on the nursing care partnership program was mailed to all 1991 clients of the Center. Fifty-five were returned. All were male, 70 percent Caucasian, 7 percent black, 7 percent Native American, 16 percent other. HIV status included 10 percent HIV only, 48 percent ARC (AIDS Related Complex), and 41 percent AIDS. Date of HIV+ diagnosis varied from 1982–1991. The following results (Table 12.4) are based on the 29 respondents who were currently in a nursing care partnership relationship at the Center.

In the second evaluation project, a convenience, nonrandomized sample of clients was surveyed regarding hospitalization and costs, use of the Center and HIV/AIDS status. For a two week period, surveys were placed in the medical treatment room and reception area, with a sign requesting clients to fill it out if they wished. All thirty respondents were male, 83 percent Caucasian, 7 percent black, 7 percent Hispanic, and 3 percent other. HIV status included 23 percent diagnosed as HIV only, 37 percent exhibiting ARC (AIDS Related Com-

Table 12.4   Nursing Care Partnership Survey Results 1991

Of the respondents in relationship with a nursing care partner (NCP), the following results were obtained:

	N = 29
I find my nursing care partner to be supportive.	100%
The NCP program helps me understand HIV/AIDS disease and my plan of treatment.	92%
The NCP program helps me negotiate the health care system.	100%
The NCP program is helpful to me.	100%

plex), and 43 percent diagnosed with full blown AIDS. Date of HIV + diagnosis varied from 1985–1992. Results (Table 12.5) are based on thirty completed surveys.

Cost Per Client Per Year Savings   The Center provides a broad range of health related services economically. Per visit costs to the Center average $65, with an average cost per client per year of $972. The costs of medical supplies and medications were not added to the Center's operating costs, because each referring hospital supplies these items for individual clients. Center clients are charged only for medically supportive treatments done there, and these treatments are billed through the clients' referring institution. Reimbursement is applied to that institution, not the Center. In addition to medically supportive treatments, clients are eligible for nursing care partner consultation, meals once a week, psychiatric and medical clinical nurse specialist consultation, massage, therapeutic touch, relaxation therapies, and Reiki treatments. Educational programs are continuously offered on symptom and disease management, prevention of complications, home care and safer sex practices. They also offer various support groups, aerobics, dental screenings, and paid employment.

Savings Realized Through Donations/Volunteer Services   In 1991, contributions to the Center in cash donations, meals, furnishings, volunteer professional and nonprofessional services equaled $52,000. These donations represent a savings of $52,000 which would otherwise have been budgeted for client services. Because of the Center's reputation as a professional nurse-managed caring center, donations and vol-

Table 12.5   Client Cost Effectiveness Survey Results

Frequency of Hospitalization:	$N = 30$
Hospitalized in last two years for complications of HIV/AIDS.	53%
Hospitalized 1–3 times in last two years.	47%
Hospitalized 4 or > times in last two years.	6%
Not hospitalized in last two years.	47%
Cost Effectiveness of Center:	
The Center teaches me self-help skills which keep me out of the hospital.	93%
The Center is important in my physical and emotional wellness.	100%
I come to the Center with symptoms before visiting a hospital or physician.	70%
I consult with my nursing care partner before requesting medical intervention.	83%
I prefer to have medical treatments done at the Center rather than a hospital.	97%
The services of the Center decrease my hospital costs.	43%

unteer support services, both professional and nonprofessional, are common.

Community and Professional Education Services   The educational and community service role of nurses has historically comprised a large part of professional nursing practice. In 1991, the Center nurses, staff and clients performed 84 presentations to more than 2,000 people, including students, professionals, and lay persons. In addition, more than 500 people visited the Center in 1991, and these visitors were comprised of health professionals, the media, hospital administrators, community and student groups. Many professionals visited the Center in order to learn how to set up a similar outpatient center elsewhere. Although a monetary cost savings figure is impossible to determine, all of these services that are a part of the Center's mission result in decreased direct, nonpersonal costs of HIV/AIDS care.

Benefits to Supporting Agencies

Although the Center is supported (in addition to its federal grant) by three hospitals, a regional AIDS Educational Training Center and the

Table 12.6 Benefits of the Denver Nursing Project in Human Caring to Supporting Institutions

BENEFITS	SUPPORTING INSTITUTIONS		
	School of Nursing	Hospitals	AIDS Educational Training Center
Innovative Clinical Practice Model	X	X	
Testing and Evaluation of Caring Theory	X		
Public Relations: Attraction of RNs/students	X	X	X
Role modeling of nursing theory based HIV/AIDS care	X	X	X
HIV/AIDS clinical research site	X		
Decreased medical costs per AIDS patient		X	
Increased patient satisfaction		X	
Improved public image: support of caring for persons with HIV		X	X

Table 12.6   Continued

BENEFITS	SUPPORTING INSTITUTIONS		
	School of Nursing	Hospitals	AIDS Educational Training Center
Association with federal grant	X		
Partial fulfillment of educative/ community service mission	X	X	X

University of Colorado School of Nursing, all of these institutions receive benefits in return. These benefits are outlined in Table 12.6.

QUALITATIVE RESEARCH REGARDING COST SAVINGS OF THE CENTER

Several qualitative methods were used to explore cost effectiveness of the Center. These included analysis of written documentation in nursing care records concerning cost savings, qualitative analysis of interviews of clients and nurses regarding the impact of the Center on health care costs, and recording of client's written comments on cost surveys. When clients and nurses were also asked to tell the researcher stories of nursing care partnership relationships, instances of cost savings emerged from the narratives. Excerpts from the stories follow (Schroeder & Maeve, 1992). All of these methods will be briefly discussed.

Nursing Care Record Documentation: Cost Effective Interactions with Clients

In addition to the above client surveys, for a four-month period in 1992 nurses kept a written log of client interactions that they felt saved hos-

Table 12.7   Nursing Care Record Documentation: Cost Effective Nursing Services

Outpatient medical treatments: Pentamidine treatments, blood transfusions, lab work, IV fluids and medications, IV site care, etc.
Nursing assessment and management of symptoms/referrals.
Provision of emotional support/support groups/counseling regarding living wills, suicide attempts.
Help with problem solving, facilitation of decision-making ability of clients.
Education regarding home care, caregiver support to maintain clients at home during periods of illness.
Education regarding nutrition, exercise, stress management, safer sex, relationships.

pital inpatient costs. These logs were matched to written documentation in the nursing care record to ascertain actual instances of cost saving services. The most recurring nursing care record entries are recorded in Table 12.7.

Client and Nurse Interviews

As part of this project on costs, clients and nurses were recently interviewed regarding their views on the impact of the Center on health care costs. Six nurses and five members of the Client Advisory Committee (an elected board of clients who provide direction to the Center's operations) were interviewed. Results were analyzed qualitatively. Major categories and comments from clients and nurses follow.

Client Comments

Emotional supportive services, caring atmosphere, nursing care partnership relationships:

> "Before I came to the Center, I had no idea where to go or what to do."

"When I was diagnosed, I felt like a freak—is there anybody else like me? Then I came to the center and people are like me here. I'm HIV positive, but I'm treated like an equal."

"I'm treated like an equal here—the hugs, someone to talk to, learning about HIV. I don't know what I'd do without the Center."

"They *listen* here, more than the docs or clinics do."

"They recognize you here, and are concerned where you are."

"I don't know what I'd do without the Center, it's like a family here."

"The Caring Center has been a place for me to come to get medical treatment and support and not worry about bigotry."

Peer support and facilitation of life style changes to a healthy lifestyle:

"When I'm able to help another physically, emotionally, or morally, it helps keep me healthy. I know it."

". . . it helps to see people 'get on with their lives' while living with HIV/AIDS; watching other people solving problems and issues helps before the desperate stage."

"I was able to quit drinking; because I no longer go to bars for social events, I'm able to be at the Center whenever I want. The nursing Center helped me make positive changes in my life."

"The aerobics class has improved my health physically and emotionally, reducing colds, neurotic activity, and clumsiness. Now I need less care."

Education for self care, preventing complications, managing symptoms, negotiating health care systems:

"Nurses tell us about symptoms, what to do, and that avoids hours waiting for doctors. They also are able to get us right in to see a doctor if we need it."

"I like knowing about symptoms, being able to just sit and talk about problems."

"The expertise and caring of the nurses teaches us how to take care of ourselves."

Use of the Center in Lieu of Physician:

"I like having Pentamidine done here, and it avoids hospital costs."

"I come here for information, rather than visiting the general medicine or psychiatric departments of the hospital.

"The Center saves some medical expenses, because I get my questions answered here rather than by a doctor or emergency room."

"There is no waiting here; I'd be fired (from my job) if I tried to walk into an Infectious Disease Clinic to be seen, because I'd wait all day."

Information From Nurses

Nursing Care Partnerships/Emotional Support:

"There is an intangible thing that occurs in caring for another person—if you care for me or believe in me, then I can do more."

"Clients call here first before calling a doctor, and assessment is done to decide if they need to be seen by a physician."

"A family member called me today about a client in the hospital— they trust us here, in the hospital they wouldn't call anyone . . . There is a level of trust here."

"(Regarding psychiatric admissions) . . . when someone is feeling borderline they come here before they go to the emergency department. Sometimes that's all they need, to feel safe . . . They come here and put things back into perspective."

Education of Client and Caregiver for Self-Care Maintain Client at Home during Periods of Illness:

"We educate people regarding disease processes and what is in their power—they have the ability to take control, circumventing learned helplessness that is present in the health care system. When people have information, they are better able to take care of themselves."

"Doctors don't communicate 'I'm sorry, I simply do not know what's going on.' I teach clients that "symptom management" will happen a lot. I say, 'I'm sorry, you can't find the answer but we can do these ten things which will help.'"

"The clients say 'The doctor won't talk to me.' I taught one client to role play with the doctor. He said he felt more control just by role playing."

"I teach everybody. My focus is promotion—at the hospital, a blood draw is just a blood draw . . . Here, it's more than that, psychosocial and physical symptoms have to be picked up on . . . (in addition to the blood draw)."

Prevention of Physician and Hospital Usage/Pooling of Health Care Resources to Save Costs:

"We reduce the cost of clients taking little problems to emergency rooms. In ER, they take up space in an already stressed system, necessitating triage and treatment."

"All medical care done here is cost effective. Sometimes the doctor doesn't need to be involved, the nurse makes decisions."

"We circumvent hospital admissions and get things done with home care."

"Pooling of resources increases productivity of nurses . . . we do a select group of procedures and we do them more often."

"Because we're here, the patients use us instead of the emergency room. For example, we discover dehydration, give them two liters at the Center, and send them home. Otherwise, they may have to wait (to be seen in a clinic or office), to their detriment."

"The three supporting institutions benefit from the efforts here, for if each institution had to run its own center, the costs would increase."

Qualitative Comments of Clients on Cost Effectiveness Survey

On the client survey of hospital costs done this year, clients were asked to describe ways the Center reduced costs if they if they agreed that the Center has a positive impact on costs. Forty-three percent of clients indicated that the Center directly reduced inpatient costs. Their comments are listed in Table 12.8.

Nurse and Client Stories: Nursing Care Partnerships and Costs

In 1991, in an attempt to further understand the experience of HIV/AIDS, a qualitative project was done which elicited client and nurse

Table 12.8   Client Comments on Cost Effectiveness Survey   1992

The Center "helps me maintain an acceptable degree of sanity" and "outlines medical treatments."

"The Center has helped me a lot with dealing with HIV, and I get a good strong feeling of support from everyone here."

"I really appreciate the level of caring and genuine kindness I receive from the nurses."

"The Center helps by reducing stress, both mental and physical."

"The support of the staff that understands the situation has been really important to mental health."

"I can have therapy done at the Center that would have to be done at the hospital."

"The Center keeps me 'weller' so (I have) less medical visits, which reduces overall expenses."

"Due to the therapy—massage, counselling, information available, approachability of the staff, knowledge—the Center has circumvented many things which could have been problems."

"I have been able to reduce my stress level and increase my physical condition through my personal involvement with the Center and therefore have not been hospitalized for an opportunistic infection. The Center not only offers outpatient treatments but also opportunities for maintenance of health and preventative education."

"The Center RNs help me stay home, not in the hospital. Symptoms are evaluated by RNs at the Center rather than in a hospital."

"At the Center I am able to ask a nurse about early symptoms that I am having, and through her help I can get an early treatment to prevent me waiting until I am too sick and need to be hospitalized."

"Many times I see a nurse about my symptoms before I see a doctor."

"I have largely depended on staff for emotional support, printed materials on nutrition and health care. I particularly appreciate the technical superiority of the nurses' blood-drawing skills."

"I feel overwhelmed with joy for a place like this. It is advantageous because of the caring, nurses and the journey we are all on."

narratives about living and working with HIV/AIDS. Although determination of cost effectiveness was not a goal of the project, instances of actual and potential inpatient cost savings emerged from the interviews. Excerpts from the interviews follow (Schroeder & Maeve, 1992).

Client: "C. was my guardian angel and probably will be again. She gives me perspective, something that is hard with AIDS. You never know if the fever will be anything, because to ignore a strange symptom sometimes means horrible things. C. knows me and can see me through a lot of things that I may have had to go to the hospital for. I feel strongly about how much the nursing center can do for us and to save money and resources. Before, I had nobody to turn to. . . . She helps me review all my options, helps me handle things myself."

Nurse: "I think the NCP (Nursing Care Partnerships) program helps avoid unnecessary emergency room visits. Often the clients are extremely anxious and don't know whether to trust their perceptions or not. Calling and talking to me is like somebody "holding" the disease for them for a while. . . . The NCP program is important for this population, we empower them to know what to ask for, to know what is good care. We teach them the information they need before they go into crisis, and teach them to manage their own care in the hospital."

Psychiatric Clinical Nurse Specialist: "I think my work with families (primarily mothers) of clients keeps clients out of institutions, because if the family is empowered to care for their children, everybody can get what they need. The ill child can die in a supportive, caring environment at home, and the family can lovingly care for the child throughout the process. . . . It often happens that a son has to move back home, sick, no job or insurance, and has to tell parents things they are not prepared for or willing to hear—not only must he tell them of this homosexuality or drug abuse, but that he has AIDS. It is extremely difficult for both parents and children; a lot of autonomy is lost on both sides. My work is to get families to talk to each other. It's tough, both sides are often angry and confused. But the rewards for all of us are worth it."

CONCLUSION

This project used quantitative and qualitative methods to explore the impact of a nurse-managed outpatient center for persons living with HIV/AIDS on health care costs. The potential cost impact of the Center is significant due to the nurses' ability to obviate hospital admissions, decrease prolonged lengths of stay, provide outpatient medically supportive treatments, care for clients at a low cost per client per year, and attract professional and nonprofessional volunteer services and donations. Perhaps more importantly, the Center's positive impact on quality of life for persons living with HIV/AIDS has been demonstrated through several evaluation research projects done in the last two years. No attempt has been made to quantify the diminished human suffering that results from a caring relationship, although clients and nurses have consistently considered this aspect the most important asset of the Center (Schroeder & Neil, 1992).

The chronic and progressive nature of HIV/AIDS, coupled with the emotional and social costs of living with a terminal and infectious disease, make apparent the fact that inpatient hospital care is not the most effective nor even the most viable option for persons living with the disease. Considering that the Center has recorded over 14,000 visits since 1988, and has been estimated to have saved over $700,000 in hospital charges for HIV/AIDS care in the last year, it is apparent that the ability of the Center to reduce overall emotional, physical, and monetary costs of HIV/AIDS is considerable.

REFERENCES

Barnes, D. (1992). A numbers game: Estimating HIV-1 infections. *The Journal of NIH Research, 4*(7), p. 10.

Community Nursing Centers gaining ground as solution to health issues. (1992). *The American Journal of Nursing, 6,* 70–71.

Fuerst, M. (1991). Cost analysis of HIV/AIDS outpatient services: Cheaper, but will they be used by IUVDS? *AIDS Patient Care, 2,* 31–33.

Green, W. (1991). The costs of AIDS in Colorado. Report prepared for the Governor's AIDS Coordinating Council, prepared by Center for Health Ethics and Policy, Graduate School of Public Affairs, University of Colorado at Denver.

Neil, R., & Schroeder, C. (1992). Evaluation research within a human caring framework. In D. Gaut (Ed.), *The presence of caring in nursing*. New York: National League for Nursing Press.

Nurse-run centers prove that good care can cost less. (1992). *American Journal of Nursing, 7,* 70–71.

Schroeder, C., & Maeve, M. (1992). Nursing care partnerships at the Denver Nursing Project in Human Caring: An application and extension of caring theory in practice. *Advances in Nursing Science, (15)* 2, 25–38.

Schroeder, C., & Neil, R. (1992). Focus groups: A humanistic means of evaluating an HIV/AIDS center. *Journal of Clinical Nursing, (1),* 265–274.

The Denver Post. AIDS treatment tab soars: Lifetime of care now costs $102,000. (July 23, 1992).

Watson, J. (1985a) *Nursing: The philosophy and science of human caring.* Boulder, CO: The Colorado Associated University Press.

Watson, J. (1985b). *Nursing: Human science and human care.* Norwalk, CO: Appleton-Century-Crofts.

Watson, J. (1988). New dimensions of human caring theory. *Nursing Science Quarterly.* (4): 175–181.

Watson, J. (1990). Transpersonal caring: A transcendent view of the person, health, and healing. In M. Parker, (Ed.), *Nursing Theories in Practice.* New York: The National League for Nursing Press.

Part VII

Martha Rogers' Theoretical Framework
for Nursing

13

Kaleidoscoping in Life's Turbulence: From Seurat's Art to Rogers' Nursing Science

Howard Karl Butcher

Nursing is an art; and, if it is to be made an art, requires an exclusive a devotion, as hard a preparation, as any painter's or sculptor's work; for what is the having to do with dead canvas or cold marble, compared with having to do with the living body—the temple of God's spirit? It is one of the Fine Arts; I had almost said, the finest of the Fine Arts. [*]

—Florence Nightingale

Ever since Nightingale, art has been a rich metaphor for nursing scholars' theoretical explanations and analyses of the essential nature of nursing. Nursing is an art form, not identical to, but rather has elements in common with other art forms, such as the performing arts of dance and music and the visual arts of painting and sculpture (Peplau, 1988). The art of nursing is its compassionate, imaginative, transforming, creative, and empowering service toward the health and well-being of humankind. The very essence of the fine arts and the art of nursing lies in their creative imagination, sensitive spirit and intelligent understanding (Stewart, 1929). Furthermore, Bronowski (1965, p. 16) states that "science is nothing else than the search for unity in the wild vari-

---

[*]See Una and the Lion in *Good Words*, © 1868, pp. 360–366.

ety of nature or . . . in the variety of our experiences. Poetry, painting, the arts are the same search."

It is not surprising, considering the links of nursing to the fine arts, that the fine arts of dancing, painting, composing music, and sculpting can serve as a rich source for original concepts relevant to the imaginative and creative development of nursing science. The development of theory relevant to guiding nursing practice is the most crucial task currently facing nursing. This paper describes the theoretical development of an original concept inspired by the fine art of painting. The concept of *kaleidoscoping* originates in Georges Seurat's neo-impressionist paintings. Rogers' (1970, 1980, 1986, 1987, 1988, 1990a, 1990b, 1992) science of unitary human being provides the conceptual frame of reference for creating conceptual meaning of kaleidoscoping within a unique nursing science perspective. Each of the subconcepts of kaleidoscoping will be conceptualized within Rogers' building blocks, principles, and supporting theories. Lastly, a practice methodology is discussed in relation to kaleidoscoping.

SEURAT'S KALEIDOSCOPIC PATTERN OF COLOR AND LIGHT

The concept of kaleidoscoping is inspired by the timeless shimmering dance of turbulence emanating from Seurat's paintings. Georges Seurat (1859–1891), a pioneering French artist, created masterworks shaped by his research into theories of color and light. Seurat's unusual painting method, called "pointillism" or "divisionism," refers to a technique of applying paint in juxtaposing points, patches, dots, flicks and commas of color, both in opposition and in harmony with one another. Seurat sought to paint in "drops of light." Each dot had the weight and density of a marble, the color and luminescence of a candy ball (Schiff, 1991). By the thousands, with precise exactitude, each dot was placed in order, each affecting the neighboring dots. His methodological divisionism and strict observation of the scientific theory of colors of scientists like Michel-Eugene Chevreul and Ogden Rood, ensured a maximum of luminosity, of color intensity, and of harmony (Herbert, 1991).

When gazing at his paintings, the dance of color and light appears turbulent in nature because of the sparkling, shimmering, glittering, and vibrating effect from the pattern of colors. Gibson (1991, p. 203) describes Seurat's pattern of color and light as an "innate turbulence." In a dance of energy, the separate dots of color and light are mixed optically. The colors vibrate and change in the eye (Herbert, 1991). The canvas is a dynamic energy field manifesting a kaleidoscopic pattern of color and light.

The turbulent display of color and light in Seurat's paintings is not unlike the shifting patterns of color and light seen when looking through a kaleidoscope. When looking through a kaleidoscope, one sees continuous changing patterns of color and light brought about by the unique relationships among bits of colored glass and reflecting surfaces. As the kaleidoscope is rotated there is constant change and continuous flowing variation in form, which reveals new, creative, and innovative manifestations of the pattern. The patterns in the kaleidoscope are never the same. They are unpredictable and reflect turbulent motion.

NURSING SCIENCE PERSPECTIVE

Creating conceptual meaning provides the foundation for developing theory (Chinn & Kramer, 1991). Conceptual meaning conveys thoughts, feelings, and ideas that reflect human experience more fully than definitions. Chinn & Kramer (1991) state that creating conceptual meaning is essentially an empiric approach that draws on aesthetic, ethical, and personal knowing. In this paper, conceptual meaning is created from personal knowing, the aesthetics of Seurat's art, Rogers' nursing science, and the contemporary theories of flow (Csikszentmihalyi, 1990) and chaos (Glieck, 1987; Peat, 1991).

Disciplines are identified by the unique conceptualization of their phenomenon of concern. The conceptualization of kaleidoscoping is guided by Rogers' science of unitary human beings. Rogers' nursing science offers nursing a view of human beings, the environment, and well-being unique to the nursing discipline. Rogers (1970, 1980, 1986, 1987, 1988, 1989, 1990a, 1992) views human beings and the environment as irreducible, indivisible, pandimensional energy fields identified by pattern. The human and environmental energy fields are integral to one another and engaged in a continuous mutual, dynamic, irreducible, nonlinear process characterized by innovation, increasing diversity, and unpredictable manifestations of patterning.

Rogers has used the kaleidoscope as a metaphor to describe changing patterns. Rogers (1970, p. 62) explains that the "organization of the living system is maintained amidst kaleidoscope alterations in the patterning of systems." Rogers (1970, p. 91) further states that "pattern evolves with kaleidoscopic uncertainty coordinate with the nature of the man-environment energy exchange taking place through space-time." Within Rogers' nursing science, the kaleidoscope metaphor signifies the unpredictability of continuously changing patterns in the human/environmental mutual process.

In this paper, *kaleidoscoping is defined as the flowing with turbulent manifestations of patterning*. The definition of kaleidoscoping includes three subconcepts: turbulence, patterning, and flow. Table 13.1 illustrates the relationship between each subconcept to a specific building block and principle within Rogers' nursing science perspective.

TURBULENCE

Turbulent manifestations emerge from the dance of color and light emanating from Seurat's canvas and in the similar shifting of patterns when looking through a kaleidoscope. Turbulence is a commotion in flow that is characterized by irregular, erratic, chaotic, and unpredictable movement. The signature of turbulence is fluctuations upon fluctuations, whorls upon whorls (Gleick, 1987).

Table 13.1   Relation Between the Subconcepts of Kaleidoscoping and Rogers' Science

SUBCONCEPT	BUILDING BLOCK	PRINCIPLE
Turbulence	Pandimensionality	Helicy
Patterning	Pattern	Resonancy
Flow	Openness (mutual process)	Integrality

Rogers' (1992) concept of pandimensionality and principle of helicy provide a theoretical understanding of turbulent manifestations. Pandimensionality is defined as a "nonlinear domain without spatial or temporal attributes" (Rogers, 1992, p. 29). The principle of helicy describes the nature of change as the "continuous, innovative, unpredictable, increasing diversity of human and environmental field patterns" (Rogers, 1992, p. 31). Rogers' inclusion of "unpredictability" in the principle of helicy is consistent with a nonlinear universe described in the concept of pandimensionality and chaos theory. Chaos theory (Briggs & Peat, 1989; Gleick, 1987; Peat, 1991) is a theory of nonlinear complex systems congruent with Rogerian science which describes the turbulent fluctuations in dynamic systems (Phillips, 1991). Both chaos theory and Rogers' concept of pandimensionality describe a nonlinear universe in which everything is interconnected. In chaos theory, nonlinearity is a model for understanding turbulence (Gleick, 1987; Briggs & Peat, 1989). In a nonlinear system, there is a hidden order of connectiveness and infinite sensitivity in which small fluctuation in one area can lead to unpredictable large fluctuations anywhere else in the system.

Rogers' (1992) description of change as an unpredictable process leading to greater creativity, innovativeness, diversity, and complexity as described by the principle of helicy is consistent with chaos theory's description of turbulence as being a source of creative change inherent in the universe. Prigogine's theory of dissipative structures describes the process of chaotic change in nonlinear systems (Prigogine & Stengers, 1984). Fluctuations in complex systems lead to spontaneous and unpredictable change in the direction of increasing complexity. Chaos is the creative source of structure and life (Briggs & Peat, 1989; Prigogine & Strengers, 1984).

Turbulence is also a human experience integral to the life process of human beings. Rogers (1970, p. 101) states that "the life process may be likened to cadences—sometimes harmonic, sometimes cacophonous, sometimes dissonant; rising and falling; now fast, now slow—ever changing in a universal orchestration of dynamic wave patterns." Humans all experience traumatic, tempestuous, chaotic life events. And as they evolve through the life process, with each period of turbulent storm we weather, they are somehow enriched and grow toward a new level of complexity and understanding. Within the concept of kaleidoscoping *turbulence is defined as a dissonant commotion in the human-environmental field process characterized by chaotic and unpredictable change.*

PATTERNING

The second subconcept in kaleidoscoping is patterning. In Seurat's paintings, pattern flowing from the canvas emerges from the shimmering and vibrating dance of color and light. Kaleidoscopes are instruments creating a continuous, nonrepeating, endless flow of changing patterns of color and light. Periodically, there are sudden total shifts in the pattern, creating an entirely new pattern of color and light. The sudden shift reflects a turbulent change in the pattern.

Pattern is a central building block in Rogers' conceptual system. Rogers (1970) describes pattern as dynamic, unitary, rhythmical, evolutionary, and "kaleidoscopic" in nature. Pattern is an abstraction that reveals itself through its manifestations. Manifestations of patterning emerge out of the human-environment mutual process. Field patterns demonstrate increasing variation and continual change. The nature of unitary field patterning is unpredictable and creative (Rogers, 1990). The principle of resonancy describes the patterning process as a continuous change from lower to higher wave frequency in human and environmental fields.

In human beings, patterns display themselves as nonrepeating rhythms in human behavior. It is through pattern manifestations that changes in energy fields are experienced, and provide clues to what the pattern is like. Within the concept of kaleidoscoping *patterning characterizes the nature of change in the mutual human/environmental field process.* Changing manifestations of patterning signify the ways in which individuals experience the world and the actions they take in their life situations. Kaleidoscopic patterns specify turbulent patterning. Turbulent life events are manifested by cacophonous, dissonant, dysynchronous, chaotic wave frequency patterns.

FLOW

Flow is the final subconcept in kaleidoscoping. Flow is most closely associated with Rogers' concept of mutual process and principle of integrality. The principle of integrality is defined as the "continuous mutual human field and environmental field process" (Rogers, 1990). The human and environmental fields are continuously open to one another and therefore, inseparable. Mutual process describes the nature of flow within human/environmental integrality. Mutual process signifies the dynamic interconnectiveness of everything. The human and environmental fields co-evolve together as they flow through and pattern one another. Flow is a characteristic of the integrality of the human and environmental energy fields.

Csikszentmihalyi's (1990) flow model, while not entirely congruent with Rogers' ontology, is useful in further explicating the nature of flow as conceptualized in kaleidoscoping. Flow illustrates the integrality and openness of human and environmental fields. Flow is a process of total involvement (Csikszentmihalyi, 1990, p. xi). Flow describes optimal experiences which are rich, meaningful, happy, and pleasurable epiphanies in the life process of human beings. Flow is a subjective state characterized by feelings of enjoyment, concentration, and deep involvement. Flow is "what a painter feels when the colors on the canvas begin to set a magnetic tension with each other, and a new thing, a living form, takes shape in front of the astonished creator" (Csikszentmihalyi, 1990, p. 3). Aesthetic enjoyment from viewing a piece of fine art, can lead to a sense of unfolding discovery through flow (Csikszentmihalyi & Robinson, 1990). Flow is associated with the experiences of playing chess, climbing mountains, composing music, and numerous other activities that people participate in not because they expect a reward after the activity is concluded, but because they enjoy what they are doing to the extent that experiencing the activity becomes its own reward. The pleasure of participating in the continuous changing patterns of a kaleidoscope can create a sense of flow. Today, some movie theaters still show changing kaleidoscopic patterns for entertainment before the start of the motion picture. The experiential consequences of deep and autotelic involvements is an intense enjoyment characterized by feelings of personal wholeness, a sense of discovery, and a sense of human connectedness (Csikszentmihalyi & Robinson, 1990).

Flow experiences do not only occur when one is totally absorbed in pleasurable activities. In periods of extreme adversity, Solzhenitsyn, Frankl, and Bettelheim have described how they transformed the most degrading experiences into flow experiences. Csikszentmihalyi (1990) states that the key to turning one's life into a unified flow experience is through a process of creating meaning in life's experiences. Meaning is created by cultivating purpose, forging resolve, and recovering harmony.

Flow is an integrating experience. Following a flow experience, the organization of the human field is more complex, differentiated, integrated and diverse. "After each experience of flow a person becomes more of a unique individual, less predictable, possessed of rarer skills" (Csikszentmihalyi, 1990, p. 41). Flow transforms a sense of chaos into a sense of harmony and order. In the course of the life process of human beings, flow experiences provide a sense of participation in the content of life and join all experience into a meaningful pattern.

In the concept of kaleidoscoping, "flowing with" refers to a process of total involvement in times of turbulent change. *Flow is intense harmonious involvement in the human-environmental field mutual process.* Flowing with patterns of turbulence facilitates knowing participation in change through the enhancement of the participant's awareness, choices, freedom to act intentionally, and intense involvement in the change process. Through the process of kaleidoscoping, the person can transform chaotic, unpredictable, traumatic, turbulent life events into opportunities for growth, self-actualization, creativity, and harmony.

KALEIDOSCOPING AS A PRACTICE METHODOLOGY

The evolution of nursing as a scientific discipline is predicated on the development of innovative research and practice methods congruent with the ontology of nursing's conceptual systems. There is a clarion call within the nursing discipline for the development of research and practice methodologies consistent with philosophical and theoretical perspectives (Parse, 1990; Phillips, 1990; Newman, 1990). Science-based nursing practice is the creative use of substantive nursing knowledge to facilitate patterning of well-being for the purpose of human betterment. The focus of nursing practice is on irreducible person's integral with the environmental (Rogers, 1992). "Promotion of well-being is the purpose of nursing" (Rogers, 1983, p. 1). Andersen & Smereck's (1989, 1992) explication of well-being based on Aristotle's (1984) theory of ethics is a useful conceptualization of well-being congruent with the conceptualization of kaleidoscoping.

Well-being is a sense of happiness, satisfaction, and peace which is attained through the vigorous seeking of excellence. The active pursuit of excellence involves the devotion of energy toward the development of skills, talents, and abilities to create personal achievements. Persons take action toward the development of unique potentialities and self-improvement no matter what the circumstances that enhance well-being (Aristotle, 1984; Andersen & Smereck, 1989, 1992). A sense of well-being is also enhanced through flow (Csikszentmihalyi, 1990).

The practice methodology associated with kaleidoscoping is adapted from Csikszentmihalyi's (1990) flow model and is organized by Barrett's (1988) Rogerian practice method. The first phase of Barrett's (1988) Rogerian practice model, pattern manifestation appraisal, is the continuous process of identifying manifestations of the human/environmental field that relate to current health events (Barrett, 1988). The second phase, deliberative mutual patterning, refers to the continuous process whereby the nurse with the client patterns the environmental field to promote harmony and well-being related to health events (Barrett, 1988) based on mutually identified patterning strategies designed to assist people to participate knowingly in change. Nurses are concerned with assisting clients with their knowing participation in change. Clients are viewed as health seekers concerned with the quality of their lives and searching for the means and ways of making health related changes. Knowing participation in change is facilitated by helping clients become more aware of their situation, more aware of their options and choices, empowering the freedom to act intentionally, and become involved in creating changes (Barrett, 1989).

Turbulent life events are integral to the life process of human beings. Turbulent events are chaotic in nature, unpredictable, and transformative. As transformative events, turbulent life experiences are a continuous source for change, creativity, and growth in the evolutionary life process of human beings. Nurses are in frequent contact with persons experiencing turbulent life events. Turbulent disruptions in harmonious human/environmental field patterning are present in persons experiencing illness. Kaleidoscoping is concerned with the flowing of a client's human field with a turbulent environmental energy field associated with a turbulent health event. When caring for a client who is experiencing turbulent life change, the nurse also kaleidoscopes with the client's chaotic field pattern.

PATTERN MANIFESTATION APPRAISAL

Initially, the nurse engages with the client's energy field by creating a climate of freedom and openness. Flowing with the client's turbulence involves intense and active harmonious participation with the client's field pattern. A rhythm and flow is established through the expression of unconditional love, compassion, and empathy. Pattern manifestation appraisal involves focusing on the experiences, perceptions and expressions of the health situation revealed through a rhythmic flow of dialogue and communion. The nurse relies on multiple modes of awareness in apprehending pattern manifestations. Intuition and tacit knowing are pandimensional modes that enable seeing of the whole, uncovering hidden patterns, and deepening the understanding of the client's experiences, perceptions, and expressions.

Pattern information has meaning only when conceptualized within a unitary context (Cowling, 1990). A unitary context refers to conceptualizing pattern information as manifestations of pattern emerging from a pandimensional human/environmental mutual process. Thus, experiences, perceptions, and expressions are inseparable from context. Pattern information being understood as pandimensional means that information is beyond the constraints of space and time. A past turbulent experience can be as real today as yesterday, and fear of an imagined event in the future is experienced in the infinite now. A current turbulent event resonates with all previous and future turbulent life events.

Together, the client and nurse mutually explore the meanings, images, symbols, metaphors, thoughts, insights, intuitions, memories, apprehensions, feelings, wishes, and imagination associated with the health situation and mutually construct a field pattern profile. The field pattern profile is inferred from the pattern information and reflects the essence of the client's experience, perception and expression of the health situation (Cowling, 1990; Martin, Forchuk, Santopinto & Butcher, 1992). The field pattern profile is usually in a narrative form, but it may be expressed in a diagram, poem, listing, phrase, or even one word. The nurse validates the mutually constructed field pattern profile by sharing the profile with the client. Cowling (1990) states that sharing the pattern appraisal with the participant is consistent with knowing participation in change. Further reflection may lead to additional pattern information and is a means of increasing the client's understanding and meaning of the experience.

DELIBERATIVE MUTUAL PATTERNING

Kaleidoscoping is flowing with turbulent manifestations of patterning. In deliberative mutual patterning (Barrett, 1988), the nurse and client discuss options that facilitate the client's ability to kaleidoscope knowingly with the turbulent process of change. In discussing how chaotic events can be transformed into "enjoyable challenges" and "harmony,"

Csikszentmihalyi (1990) presents three steps that are involved in the transformation of turbulence into potential flow experiences: cultivating purpose, forging resolve, and recovering harmony. Purpose, resolution, and harmony unify life and give it meaning by transforming it into a seamless flow experience (Csikszentmihalyi, 1990).

In cultivating purpose during deliberative mutual patterning, clients identify personal goals. In order to cultivate purpose one must have clear goals to strive for (Csikszentmihalyi, 1990). Setting personal goals is associated with the recognition of challenges, developing skills, and developing a system of action. The nurse participates in the client's health patterning by assisting clients identify goals that are meaningful to their own sense of well-being. Goal setting is a mutual process. The nurse does not impose her own value system by setting goals for the client, rather the nurse empowers client's knowing participation in change by facilitating clients in identifying their own goals.

Cultivating purpose includes choosing and developing an "action system." When experiencing turbulence, persons often feel immobilized. The action system consists of mutually identified strategies designed for the actualization of goals. Actualization of goals facilitates the possibility of achieving maximum well-being within one's potential.

Often a client's perceptual field is so constricted in turbulent times that they have difficulty visualizing the whole of the situation. "Creative suspension" facilitates the visualizing and understanding of the whole unfolding situation (Peat, 1991). The nurse can use guided imagery as a means to help clients initially enter a timeless suspension which enables seeing the whole and potentiates the creation of new solutions. Creative solutions are then incorporated into a personalized action system.

In order to accomplish flow in turbulent times, client's may need assistence in becoming deeply involved in the chosen system of action (Csikszentmihalyi, 1990). Forging resolve requires full immersion in the action system. Peat (1991) points out that systems in turbulence require "gentle action." Chaotic systems are infinitely sensitive. Entering a chaotic system with a "big splash" will only increase the perturbations. It is not possible to manage or steer a chaotic system in a conventional fashion because of its infinite sensitivity. Rather than trying to force a chaotic system in a particular direction, one has to act globally throughout the system (Peat, 1991). "Gentle actions" are subtle actions distributed over the whole system and are an extension of creative suspension (Peat, 1991). To live in the heart of chaos involves constantly making vanishingly small but globally coordinated movements in harmony accelerating change. The nurse can assist clients in creating "ripples" which are global gentle actions directed toward the smoothing of turbulent human/environmental field patterns. Gentle actions are the pandimensional creative solutions to weathering difficult times.

Murphy (1992) lists what he calls "integral practices" which are designed to cultivate physical, vital, affective, cognitive, volitional, and transformative dimensions of human functioning in an integrated way. Cultivating creativity, courage, balance, calm, and resilience in the midst of turbulent or threatening circumstances through deliberative mutual patterning strategies potentially enhances kaleidoscoping. Creativity can be nurtured through small group processes; exposure to fantasy science fiction, or other literature that reconceptualizes ordinary experiences; brainstorming activities; and meditation and guided imagery experiences (Murphy, 1992). Courage can be developed by transforming fear through group support; self-reflection; catharsis; and physical exercise that facilitates a sense of well-being. Balance and calm can be developed through contemplative prayer; dance and sports that promote grace under pressure; and physical exercise that promotes steadiness of the human field (Murphy, 1992). Resilience can be enhanced through self-reflection that is directed toward hopeful yet realistic perspectives on life. These are just some of the possible strategies nurses can utilize with clients experiencing turbulent life events. It is important that the choice of patterning strategies are individualized and made by the clients themselves.

Sustained gentle improvement requires paying attention and understanding the whole of what is occurring. Nurses can assist clients in concentrating on the experience through focusing exercises. Focusing is also a sustained process of systematically contacting the more central meanings of an experience (Moustakas, 1990). Creating meaning involves bringing order to the experience by synthesizing one's gentle actions into a unified flow experience. The nurse focuses on assisting the client in uncovering the hidden personal meanings in the turbulent life event. The discovery of new knowledge, increasing diversity, and self-actualization emerges from finding meaning in a turbulent life event.

The potential consequence of forging life by purpose and resolution is a sense of harmony (Csikszentmihalyi, 1990). The nurse can guide the client toward recovering harmony by exploring the positive aspects of change thereby facilitating more enjoyment in the immediate experience. Harmony can be sustained by mutually identifying flow activities that can be incorporated into the client's daily activities. Art, music, exercise, reading, gardening, meditation, dancing, sports, sailing, swimming, carpentry, sewing, and yoga are some of the many potential flow activities.

The art of sciencing is a creative process. Art and science reveal themselves as simply the left and right hands of a single process of discovery (Johnston, 1984/1986). Literature, poetry, art, music, dance, drama, cinema, and photography all hold tremendous potential as a source for new concepts for nursing theory construction. Nursing is an aesthetic experience. The art of kaleidoscoping with turbulence, as in the fine arts, is a creative expression of beauty and grace. Beauty fills us with passion; it graces us with joy and lights up our existence. A landscape, a piece of music, a film, a dance—suddenly all dreariness is gone, we are left bewitched, we are dazzled (Serrucci, 1990). Beauty brightens the darkness of despair, and with its colorful spontaneity, it regenerates nurses' lives and the lives of those who benefit from nursing care.

REFERENCES

Andersen, M. D., & Smereck, G. A. D. (1992). The consciousness rainbow: An explication of Rogerian field pattern manifestations. *Nursing Science Quarterly, 5*, 72–79.

Andersen, M. D., & Smereck, G. A. D. (1989). Personalized nursing LIGHT model. *Nursing Science Quarterly, 2*, 120–130.

Aristotle (1984). Metaphysics. In J. Barnes (Ed.). *The Complete Works of Aristotle*. Princeton, NJ: Princeton University Press.

Barrett, E. A. M. (1988). Using Rogers' science of unitary human beings in practice. *Nursing Science Quarterly, 2*, 50–51.

Barrett, E. A. M. (1989). A nursing theory of power for nursing practice: Derivation from Rogers' paradigm. In J. Riehl-Sisca (Ed.). *Conceptual models for nursing practice*. (Third Edition.) Norwalk, CT: Appleton & Lange.

Barrett, E. A. M. (1990). Rogerian patterns of scientific inquiry. In E. A. M. Barrett (Ed.). *Visions of Rogers' science-based nursing*. New York: National League for Nursing Press.

Briggs, J., & Peat, F. D. (1989). *Turbulent mirror: An illustrated guide to chaos theory and the science of wholeness*. New York: Harper & Row.

Bronowski, J. (1965). *Science and human values*. New York: Julian Messner.

Carboni, J. T. (1991). A Rogerian theoretical tapestry. *Nursing Science Quarterly, 4,* 130–136.

Chinn, P. L., & Kramer, M. K. (1991). *Theory and nursing: A systematic approach*. St. Louis: Mosby.

Csikszentmihalyi, M. (1990). *Flow: The psychology of optimal experience*. New York: Harper & Row.

Csikszentmihalyi, M., & Robinson, R. E. (1990). *The art of seeing: An interpretation of the aesthetic encounter*. Malibu, CA: The J. Paul Getty Trust.

Cowling, W. R. (1990). A template for unitary pattern-based nursing practice. In E. A. M. Barrett (Ed.). *Visions of Rogers' science-based nursing*. New York: National League for Nursing Press.

Gibson, M. (1991). Georges Seurat: Precocious genius. *The World & I, 10,* 200–205.

Gleick, J. (1987). *Chaos: Making a new science*. New York: Penguin Books.

Herbert, R. L. (1991). *Georges Seurat (1859–1891)*. New York: The Metropolitan Museum of Art, Harry N. Abrams, Inc.

Johnston, C. M. (1984/1986). *The creative imperative: Human growth & planetary evolution*. Berkeley, CA: Celestial Arts.

Martin, M., Forchuk, C., Santopinto, M., & Butcher, H. K. (1992). Alternative approaches to nursing practice: Application of Peplau, Rogers, and Parse. *Nursing Science Quarterly, 5,* 80–85.

Moustakas, C. (1990). *Heuristic research: Design, methodology and applications*. Newbury Park, CA: Sage.

Murphy, M. (1992). *The future of the body: Explorations into the further evolution of human nature*. Los Angeles: Tarcher.

Newman, M. A. (1990). Newman's theory of health as praxis. *Nursing Science Quarterly, 3*, 37–41.

Nightingale, F. (1868, June 1). Una and the lion. *Good words*, 360–366.

Parse, R. R. (1990). Parse's research methodology with an illustration of the lived experience of hope. *Nursing Science Quarterly, 3*, 9–17.

Peat, F. D. (1991). *The philosopher's stone: Chaos, synchronicity, and the hidden world order.* New York: Bantam.

Peplau, H. E. (1988). The art and science of nursing: Similarities, differences, and relations. *Nursing Science Quarterly, 1*, 8–15.

Phillips, J. (1991). Chaos in nursing research. *Nursing Science Quarterly, 4*, 96–97.

Phillips, J. (1990). New methods of research: Beyond shadows of nursing science. *Nursing Science Quarterly, 3*, 1–2.

Prigogine, I., & Stengers, I. (1984). *Order out of chaos: Man's new dialogue with nature.* Boulder, CO: New Science Library.

Rogers, M. E. (1970). *An introduction to the theoretical basis of nursing.* Philadelphia: F. A. Davis.

Rogers, M. E. (1980) Nursing: A science of unitary man. In J. Riehl & C. Roy (Eds.). *Conceptual models for nursing practice.* (2nd ed.) New York: Appleton-Century-Crofts.

Rogers, M. E. (1983). *Charting the future.* Paper presented at the First National Rogerian Conference. New York University, NY.

Rogers, M. E. (1986). Science of unitary human beings. In V. M. Malinski (Ed.). *Explorations on Martha Rogers' science of unitary human beings.* Norwalk, CT: Appleton-Century-Crofts.

Rogers, M. E. (1987). Rogers' science of unitary human beings. In R. R. Parse (Ed.). *Nursing science: Major paradigms, theories, and critiques.* Toronto: Saunders.

Rogers, M. E. (1988). Nursing science and art: A prospective. *Nursing Science Quarterly, 1*, 99–102.

Rogers, M. E. (1989). Nursing: A science of unitary human beings. In

Riehl-Sisca (Ed.). *Conceptual models for nursing practice.* (3rd ed.) Norwalk, CT: Appleton & Lange.

Rogers, M. E. (1990). Nursing: Science of unitary, irreducible, human beings: Update 1990. In E. A. M. Barrett (Ed.). *Visions of Rogers' science-based nursing.* New York: National League for Nursing Press.

Rogers, M. E. (1990). Space age paradigms for new frontiers in nursing. In M. Parker, *Nursing Theories in Practice* (pp. 109–113), New York: National League for Nursing Press.

Rogers, M. E. (1992). Nursing science and the space age. *Nursing Science Quarterly, 5,* 27–34.

Schiff, B. (1991). "Let's go get drunk on light once more." *Smithsonian, 7,* 100–111.

Serrucci, P. (1990). Inevitable grace: Breakthroughs in the lives of great men and women: Guides to your self realization. Los Angeles: Parcker, Inc.

Stewart, I. M. (1929). The science and art of nursing, editorial. *Nursing Education Bulletin, 2,* 1.

14

Unitary Practice: Revisionary Assumptions

W. Richard Cowling, III

INTRODUCTION

Unitary pattern practice derived from Martha Rogers' science of unitary human beings has been the subject of two recent papers (Cowling, 1992; Cowling, 1991), a book chapter (1990) and one upcoming article (Cowling, in press). The following practice constituents were articulated and explicated in these works:

UNITARY PATTERN PRACTICE CONSTITUENTS

1. The basic referent of nursing practice is human energy field pattern.
2. Human field pattern is appraised through manifestations of the pattern in the form of experience, perception, and expressions.
3. Pattern appraisal requires an inclusive perspective of what counts as pattern information (energetic manifestations).
4. Knowledge derived from pattern information involves multiple modes of awareness by the nurse.
5. Pattern information has meaning for pattern appraisal only when constructed within a unitary context.

6. Various formats for presenting and conveying pattern appraisal are applicable to the unitary perspective.

7. The primary source for validating pattern appraisal is the client.

8. The basic foundation for mutually-derived purposive nursing strategies is knowing participation in change.

9. Evaluation methodologies are focused on continual pattern appraisal, consequences of strategies, and confirmation of alterations with the client.

The purpose of this chapter is to refine and extend the practice constituents based on experience with clients, consideration of their viability in practice, and consistency with the unitary worldview.

The Idea of Guiding Assumptions for Practice

Originally the constituents were incorporated into a template of unitary pattern-based practice (Cowling, 1990). The terms *constituent* and *template* do not convey the intent of these statements about practice. Constituents implies a conglomeration of parts or components. Template has a connotative meaning that suggests that this group of statements should be applied uniformly to all situations for accuracy. These statements were not designed to judge the accuracy of practice. These statements originally arose from the integration of a unitary worldview into the realm of practice and are consequently based on experience wedded with theoretical pondering. The phrase *guiding assumptions for practice* best reflects the intent of these statements.

The concept of assumptions for practice has been reinforced most significantly for the author by Mary Wilson Schaef in *Beyond Therapy, Beyond Science* (1992). In describing her attempt to recognize and explore the assumptions inherent in her training and worldview she came to the following conclusion: "I tried to reconcile the worldview out of which I had come with what I knew and what I was learning and experiencing. I saw how important it is to 'name' our experience and our reality. As I did this I began to question what I see as violence done in the name of science and healing in the helping professions. I began to ask if psychologists and people in the helping professions are open to asking themselves the question: Is the unspoken worldview that under-lies the assumptions from which I practice my profession perhaps, un-wittingly, contributing to the very problems I am committed to solve? If we are not open to struggling with this question and articulating our assumptions, we are, indeed, part of the problem" (p. 10). This chapter is a response to that plea and challenge for my practice view of nursing.

UNITARY PRACTICE ASSUMPTIONS

The basic referent of nursing practice is human energy field pattern. This practice assumption is meant to convey that a unitary perspective pattern is the focus because it is that which distinguishes or differentiates fields, not boundaries or parts. In other frameworks referents for prac-tice might be the functional status of the person, developmental stage, disease condition, etc. Field pattern is one of the universal building blocks of the conceptual system described by Rogers (1990).

Human field pattern is *appreciated* through manifestations of the pat-tern in the form of experience, perception, and expressions. The term appraisal implies evaluation and estimation of quality, amount, size, and other features (*American Heritage*, 1985). It was originally cho-sen because of the secondary definition related to estimating quality or features which could be applied to human field pattern. The intent of this activity from a unitary perspective is more aligned to the term appreciate. The various definitions of "appreciate" fit the intent of uni-tary nursing. These include recognizing the quality, significance, mag-nitude, or value of an entity; being fully aware of or sensitive to or realizing; being thankful or grateful for; and enjoying or understanding critically or emotionally (*American Heritage*, 1985, p. 121). Another somewhat related definition is that of raising the value or price. In a sense this may fit as well because as a nurse gets to be more fully aware of human field pattern, he or she may experience a shift in valuing of that person. In other words, the intent of appraisal is evaluating and estimating, while the intent of appreciation is recognizing and being aware of and sensitive to something.

Manifestations of human field pattern are the means of accessing the field. Humans are known by the characteristics that are exhibited in the form of manifestations of unitary pattern flowing from the inte-grality of human/environment process. Human data sources are conceptualized in this practice view as experience, perception, and expression. Humans are constantly and contiguously all-at-once experiencing, perceiving, and expressing, providing the source for human field pattern appreciation. Experience is the raw encounter with phenomena that occurs in the process of living. Experience is conceived in its broadest sense to cover all modes of awareness (Wilber, 1982). Perceiving is the apprehending of experience or the ability to reflect while experiencing. It is also the making sense of what is happening in living. Perception is also the cornerstone of "knowing participation in change" described by Rogers (1990) as within the capacity of all human beings. Expression is the making known or the setting forth. Expressing is the manifesting of experience and perceiving which is reflective of one's underlying pattern.

Pattern *appreciation* requires an inclusive perspective of what counts as pattern information (*energetic manifestations*). One of the distinctive differences between unitary nursing and other forms of nursing is attention to a wide array of phenomena relevant to pattern recognition and appreciation. Data are not divided into sets and labeled according to categories such as spiritual, physical, emotional, mental, social, cultural, and biological. Rather all data are conceived as energetic manifestations of unitary field. Further, energetic manifestations occur experientially, meaning one is capable of experiencing what one is manifesting. Like William James (cited in LeShan & Margenau, 1982, p. 44), experience is viewed as "any item or ingredient within our stream of consciousness." This is the type of inclusivity necessary to fully embrace unitary pattern.

LeShan and Margenau (1982) distinguish cognitive from noncognitive experience, unnecessary in a unitary view of practice. However, these distinctions are reinterpreted to make a point here. Cognitive experiences are those that lead to knowledge or understanding and noncognitive experiences are such phenomena as feelings, values, beauty, friendship, love, esthetic enjoyment. The experience of a house as an architectural structure is cognitive, while the experience of a house as a home is noncognitive. The important point here is not whether experiences are cognitive or noncognitive. In a unitary view it is possible that experience be accompanied simultaneously by multiple perceptual features that are integral to that experience. For instance, the above case of experiencing house and home are equally significant.

This is of critical import when we begin to move from such an example to the phenomenon we encounter as nurses in practice. Pain, for instance, is often conceptualized as both cognitive and noncognitive and treated based on this defining feature. If one views pain as experience (raw experience that does not have to be categorized) accompanied by perceptual features reflective of underlying unitary pattern, the relevance of this data form shifts. The practice of unitary pattern appreciation involves awareness and sensitivity to the unitary pattern underlying pain in its fullness rather than the differentiation of the experience as cognitive or noncognitive (for some clinicians translated as a difference between real and imagined pain).

Clearly the distinctions of experience as spiritual, psychological, and biological have no meaning in unitary terms other than to be accepted as ways humans have been taught to categorize experience for some purposes. There are those in the unitary camp who would argue for exclusion of forms of data such as blood pressure or pulse rate in accounting for unitary pattern. These data comprise unitary information by the mere fact that in a unitary view they could not be particulate; in other words, how could they be particulate when there are no parts in a unitary view. These data (called physical data by most clinicians) take on new meaning when conceptualized as energetic manifestations of a unitary field. Further, it has been demonstrated that one experiences these "physical" phenomena with or without the use of monitoring apparatus or techniques. One experiences the pounding pressure and the racing pulses to varying degrees, perhaps associated with the degree of awareness. Discounting this data source as non-unitary would be to deny acceptance of the fullest expression of unitary pattern.

Knowledge derived from pattern *appreciation* involves multiple modes of awareness by the nurse. Expressions of pattern form the informational substance for pattern appreciation by the nurse. It is through expressions of pattern that the nurse comes to derive knowledge of the underlying pattern. Tapping these expressions requires multiple modes of awareness because of the many forms that comprise the pattern expressions. Expressions include sensations reported by individuals and observed phenomenon such as gait, posture, position, activity level, muscle strength, and tears to name a few. Other examples of phenomena as expressions of unitary pattern are meditative insights, sense of oneness with all, sensations of movement or shifting change, sadness, dreams, beliefs, and concerns. In essence, anything expressed is relevant to unitary pattern since humans are unitary creatures.

A unitary view requires attention to all realms of data, including sensory data. As Michael Murphy (1992) has pointed out, "without data from many domains of inquiry, without various kinds of knowing, our understanding of human development will be incomplete" (p. 14). Likewise, for unitary nursing, to deny this data is to deny the full range of human experience and consequently, diminish the fullest appreciation of unitary pattern.

The assumptions of the unitary paradigm offer the position of a more inclusive view of experiential data and consequently the potentiality of these data to be revealed to the practitioner. This process can be compared to that of the quest for data acquisition and verification in religious life described by Wilber (1983). He makes the point that a person must be developmentally adequate to a disclosure, or there will be no disclosure. The example from religious inquiry would be with the experience of meditative knowing. The techniques of Zen are injunctive tools to that disclosure. Consequentially, the unitary view requires a responsiveness to a wider array of experiential data that is brought about by certain injunctive tools. These injunctive tools, the emerging and evolving methodologies associated with the paradigm, provide means for exposure to the phenomena. Additionally, the unitary view when committed to freely, allows for disclosure of facts unknown without it.

The inquiry processes associated with the various paradigms within nursing science are dissimilar in this regard. Although all the paradigms, or the perspectives inherent in them have rules for injunction and for appropriate disclosure of data, the underlying assumptions differentiate and guide nursing practice. An extremely important notion here is that in order to be willing to use the injunctive devices associated with a paradigm, one must have a certain openness to the potential revelation of data. Openness to the revelation of data in nursing springs from individual and consensual views on what phenomena are relevant for study.

Several nursing authors have provided potential clues to developing the necessary injunctive tools for revealing more clearly the pattern data of unitary fields. Newman (1986) has described a pattern recognition process that involves "going into ourselves and getting in touch with our own pattern and through it in touch with the pattern of the person or persons with whom we are interacting" (p. 72). Phillips (1988) described a process of uncovering human-environment patterns of wholeness through a "wedding of observable and unobservable manifestations" embodying both concreteness and abstractness (p. 96). Smith (1988) suggests the need for a "motion lens" approach to pattern recognition that would "identify configurations of the rhythmical flow in the person-environment process" (p. 94). These approaches will develop further with specified rules for injunction that reflect awareness and sensitivity to phenomena as unitary field energetic manifestations. Work already being done on intuition in nursing (Agan, 1987; Benner, 1984; Benner & Tanner, 1987; Rew, 1986; Rew & Barrow, 1987; Schraeder & Fischer, 1986) reflects both a potential unitary mode of pattern recognition and appreciation and a specification of clear rules of injunction for using intuition. This could serve as a model for further development of other approaches to unitary knowing.

A construction process of synopsis and synthesis is requisite to pattern knowing. The previous constituent assumption was, "pattern information has meaning for pattern appraisal only when constructed within a unitary context" (Cowling, 1990, p. 56). This unitary context was described as having several characteristics which also have been modified. Some of these characteristics revised from previous specifications (Cowling, 1990) are:

1. Data or information from the client (any expression of the client) is unitary and not particular.

2. Inclusion of information expressing a sensation of temporality, space, or movement is viewed as pandimensional and not linear or three-dimensional.

3. Pattern information or data does not exist separately in reality.

4. Human/environmental phenomena are integral and inseparable and use of boundaries on the human and environment are constructed.

5. Pattern information or data reflects the distinctive unitary field from which it emanates.

These distinctive characteristics of a unitary context remain of extreme importance since it is still common to confuse system and/or holistic contexts as synonymous with unitary. The specific differentiation of these contexts was explained in a recent article (Cowling, in press) which demonstrated how data or information is used in making a biopsychosocial assessment and how this same data is used for unitary pattern recognition. Biopsychosocial (holistic/system) assessment involves the separation of data into categories, looking for interrelationships among the categories, and either looking at how one data category represents other data categories (physical pain accounted for by psychological distress) or reduction of data to one data category (all behavior a result of physiological process). These assessment strategies emphasize that the behavior of the whole is different from the parts. Yet extensive data are collected on all the parts as evidenced by the lengthy assessment formats in most general nursing textbooks.

The approach to data from a unitary perspective involves synopsis and synthesis. The model for understanding data from a unitary context which has potential is the one used by Murphy (1992) based on Broad's (1953) synoptic empiricism. "Synopsis is the deliberate viewing together of aspects of human experience which, for one reason or another, are generally kept apart by the plain man and even by the professional scientist or scholar. The object of synopsis is to try to find out how these various aspects are inter-related. Synthesis is the attempt to supply a coherent set of concepts and principles which cover satisfactorily all the regions of fact which have been viewed synoptically" (p. 8).

One necessary and important modification in this model would be on the object of the synopsis. Broad's (1953) object of finding out *how* the various aspects of human experience are inter-related is more consistent with a holistic or biopsychosocial perspective. This assumes that one is searching (in Broad's case a scientist) for the relationship of parts. As noted previously, a unitary view assumes wholeness and irreducibility of the human overriding any notion of the existence of parts. In other words, the data one is dealing with are integral because humans are whole and one does not need to find out *how* these data are inter-related. Consequently, the object of synopsis from a unitary practice perspective would be to search for the clearest and fullest picture of unitary pattern that is reflected in the data or information presented to the practitioner.

The role of synthesis remains essentially the same. Synthesis seeks a coherent set of concepts and principles which cover all the data which are viewed synoptically. In a unitary practice context the purpose of synthesis requires greater specification. Synthesis would be aimed at providing concepts and principles relevant to unitary practice for a specific person. Unitary concepts and principles emerge from a specific set of synoptically viewed data from one individual. This distinction is extremely important given the original perspective espoused by Broad (1953) which focused on sets of data or findings across fields of study or multiple empirical investigations.

Various formats for presenting and conveying pattern *appreciation* are applicative to the unitary perspective. There is no singular format prescribed for conveying pattern appreciation (Cowling, 1990). Pattern appreciation reflects a synoptic view of the data for an individual client. This synoptic picture has been termed a pattern profile (Cowling, 1990). The synoptic pattern profile is used to create an image of the person's underlying field pattern as reflected in the various aspects of human experience, perceptions, and expressions presented by the individual. Therefore, the question a unitary practitioner is faced with is, "what profile form best represents an image of the underlying field pattern based on data (experience, perception, expressions)?" Potential profile forms can be one sentence or phrase, a single word, a narrative in various formats such as a story or poem, a drawing, a symbol, a configuration of words, a diagram, a selected piece of music, or an object selected or created to represent the person's pattern.

This description of creating a pattern profile does not fully convey the nature of the profiling process. Embedded in the synoptic processing of information are two significant considerations reported earlier. The first is that the practitioner must be open to and willing to accept a wide array of information as relevant to unitary pattern. The second is that the practitioner must be developmentally adequate to data or information disclosure, or there will be no disclosure. This requires the use of injunctive tools that lead to that disclosure. In summary, the practice of unitary nursing requires a responsiveness to a wider array of experiential data that is brought about by certain injunctive tools.

The primary source for *verifying* pattern *appreciation and profile* is the client. The previous assumption used the word "validating" which was inappropriate since validation pertains more to the logic of an argument (Flew, 1979, pp. 363–365) and to justification or soundness of statements (*American Heritage*, 1985, p. 1335). Verifying implies attention to the truth claim of a statement (Flew, 1979, p. 368) and to confirmation of the truth of a fact (American Heritage, 1985, p. 1343). This is a rather truncated way of saying that the unitary practitioner accepts the client's truth claim of the realness of information. Verification by the client assumes that self-knowledge is an acceptable form of information and actualizes for the practitioner in her work with the client knowing participation in change.

Verifying pattern information, and subsequently the appreciation that is shaped into a profile, is undertaken in a way which is consistent with the client's ability to understand the concept of underlying pattern. For some clients, the appreciation and profile can be spoken about in terms of experiences and perceptions related to health or a client-defined issue or topic of relevance. Observed and self-reported information is integrated into the pattern appreciation and the synthesized profile is presented to the client for verification. Another approach which has been used is to focus more directly on the pattern information and the degree to which it represents the experience, perceptions, and expressions of the client (Cowling, 1990). The profile is presented to the client and he or she might be asked if this is a good summation of the information without using the terms pattern or profile. These verification procedures are tailored to the individual and his or her responsiveness to and understanding of a unitary picture of reality.

The basic foundation for purposive nursing strategies is knowing participation in change. The original constituent used the term "intervention" (Cowling, 1990) and was subsequently altered to "mutually-derived purposive nursing strategies" (Cowling, in press). This was done because intervention implies "coming in between" two entities or periods of time and to interfere, hinder, or modify usually through force (American Heritage, 1985, p. 672). These defining characteristics are inconsistent with the unitary view of inseparable entities and acausality.

The term "mutually-derived" is dropped at this time because it has potential for misrepresenting the meaning of the assumption by detracting from what is central to unitary practice, knowing participation in change by the client. One of the most important consequences, and biggest challenges, of operating in practice from a unitary paradigm is to accommodate the human capacity for knowing participation in change. At the same time this is not a model that is based upon the passivity of the unitary practitioner. What is required of the practitioner who accepts knowing participation in change is a radical shift from the control model of traditional health practice and of helping in general.

A unitary model of practice is essentially a participatory, egalitarian model of practice. The basis for action on the part of the practitioner is the participation of the client with his or her own life process. A clear example of such a model, based on assumptions consistent with a unitary view, is the Living Process System proposed by Schaef (1992). It is impossible to fully describe this model here. It is not based upon the science of unitary human beings, but what is important is that it offers at least five important features critical to unitary practice. It advocates for practitioner receptivity to and honoring of the client's own living process. This means that the practitioner is not seen as an intervener who interferes with an inherent healing capacity of the client. The client and helper are viewed as equal participants in any helping encounter. This does not mean that the practitioner does not use knowledge and theory, but these arise from the experience itself. The hallmark feature of the model is participation in one's life process, which I would reconceptualize as one's unitary patterning. This accommodates knowing participation in change by the client. This life process model requires surrender of control usually associated with helping and healing encounters. This means giving up the traditional notion of knowing about cause and effect in order to promote change in someone else. Finally, this model denies diagnosis as the foundation of practice decisions and relies on wisdom from participation with clients. Embedded in this denial of diagnosis is a rejection of a dualistic view of reality (what is sick and not-sick) and of judgment as a critical attribute for healing to occur.

The concepts and principles of unitary practice for the individual client emerge from pattern appreciation and approaches are determined by the client. The original constituent was stated as, "evaluation methodologies are focused on continual pattern appraisal and confirmation of alterations with the client" (Cowling, 1990). Later this was altered to include, "evaluation methodologies are focused on continual pattern appraisal, *consequences of strategies*, and confirmation of alterations with the client" (Cowling, in press). This constituent assumption has been dropped altogether and replaced. The previous statement implies a linear, judgmental process of evaluation which does not fit the unitary paradigm.

The new assumption conveys the idea that the substance and actions of unitary practice are arrived at through the process of pattern appreciation. In the process of synthesis of pattern information there is an emergence of meaning from the data that reveals specific concepts relevant to individual pattern. Similarly, the principles of practice for that individual person become evident. In other words, the experiential, perceptual, and expressive data as synthesized guide the nursing for that client. Possible approaches relevant to that individual become more and more evident.

This new constituent assumption stems from a recent shift in thinking for the author that will probably shift again. Schaef (1992) depicts a similar shift for herself in which her field, psychology, encouraged the acceptance or development of theory and then operated out of it. "That approach results in a tendency to make theory static and holy. It offers security and breeds rigidity. Professionals who operate in this way become 'theory-bound.' My work informs my theory. By doing what works, by being led by the people with whom I work and not trying to fit them into my 'theory' or preconceived notions, I have been able to hear and see them and myself, and have constantly to reassess what I do and to be willing to modify endlessly" (p. 4). Further, Schaef (1992) notes the danger of limiting and controlling the practitioner's perception by theory, causing them not to hear or to dismiss information that does not support their theories. Additionally, theory may serve to take the practitioner away from the client by not allowing him or her to be present because the practitioner is so busy thinking about the theory.

The determination of approaches is within the realm of free choice. This is not only consistent with a unitary view, it is consistent with the values of a truly participatory frame of reference. The goal is to support human endeavors to knowingly participate in change of human field patterning. Unitary practice is not technique driven because techniques can often lead to inappropriate generalization from one client to another. The technique can become an imposed force for change rather than one that emerges from participating.

SUMMARY

The purpose of this chapter has been to articulate a revision of the original unitary pattern practice constituents (Cowling, 1990; 1991; 1992; in press). The constituents have been modified individually and renamed "guiding assumptions for practice" consistent with the intent of the author, the unitary worldview, and the author's experience with clients. These assumptions are shared with a community of scholar/practitioners in nursing for critique and commentary. Further, they are shared in a spirit of honesty about my own struggles to creatively use the unitary perspective with clients and to challenge all practitioners to own and name the assumptions and worldview that underlie their practice.

REFERENCES

Agan, R. D. (1987). Intuitive knowing as a dimension of nursing. *Advances in Nursing Science, 10*(1), 63–70.

American Heritage Dictionary (2nd ed.) (1985). Boston: Houghton Mifflin Company.

Benner, P. (1984). *From novice to expert*. Menlo Park, CA: Addison-Wesley.

Benner, P., & Tanner, C. (1987). How expert nurses use intuition. *American Journal of Nursing, 87*, 23–31.

Broad, C. D. (1953). *Religion, philosophy and psychical research*. New York: Harcourt, Brace.

Cosier, R. A., & Aplin, J. C. (1982). Intuition and decision making: Some empirical evidence. *Psychological Report, 5*, 275–281.

Cowling, W. R. (1990). A template for unitary pattern-based practice. In E. A. M. Barrett (Ed.), *Visions of Rogers' science-based nursing* (pp. 45–65). New York: National League for Nursing Press.

Cowling, W. R. (1991, April). *Unitary pattern-based practice*. Paper presented at Third South Florida Nursing Theorist Conference, Miami, FL.

Cowling, W. R. (1992, June). *Unitary pattern practice*. Paper presented at Fourth Rogerian Conference, New York, NY.

Cowling, W. R. (in press). Unitary knowing in nursing practice. *Nursing Science Quarterly*.

LeShan, L., & Margenau, H. (1982). *Einstein's space and Van Gogh's sky: Physical reality and beyond*. New York: Macmillan.

Murphy, M. (1992). *The future of the body: Explorations into the further evolution of human nature.* Los Angeles: Tarcher.

Newman, M. (1984). Nursing diagnosis: Looking at the whole. *American Journal of Nursing, 84,* 1496–1499.

Phillips, J. R. (1988). The looking glass of nursing research. *Nursing Science Quarterly, 1,* 96.

Rew, L. (1986). Intuition: Concept analysis of a group phenomenon. *Advances in Nursing Science, 8*(2), 21–28.

Rew, L., & Barrow, E. M. (1987). Intuition: A neglected hallmark of nursing knowledge. *Advances in Nursing Science, 10*(1), 49–62.

Rogers, M. E. (1990). Nursing: Science of unitary, irreducible, human beings: Update 1990. In E. A. M. Barrett (Ed.), *Visions of Rogers' science-based nursing* (pp. 5–11). New York: National League for Nursing Press.

Schaef, A. W. (1992). *Beyond therapy, beyond science.* New York: HarperCollins.

Smith, M. J. (1988). Perspectives of wholeness: The lens makes a difference. *Nursing Science Quarterly, 1,* 94–95.

Wilber, K. (1982). The problem of proof. *Revision: A Journal of Consciousness and Change, 5*(1), 80–100.

Part VIII

The Roy Adaptation Model

15

The Roy Adaptation Model: Theoretical Update and Knowledge for Practice

Sister Callista Roy
Carolyn Padovano Corliss

It is significant that nurses from practice settings throughout the country meet in sessions such as the South Florida Nursing Theorist Conference. The work of the past 25 years to describe the assumptions, values, and concepts of the discipline have the ultimate goal of providing direction for nursing practice. Nurses are eager for the long promised relating of theory to practice. The various theoretical approaches offer to nurses in the dramatically changing health care scene a centering point for defining nursing practice, the basis for developing knowledge for practice through research, and, in turn, the science of nursing applicable to nursing education. The Roy Adaptation Model is a particularly widely used and well developed approach to outlining the basic and clinical sciences of nursing. From this paradigm view, one can address today's practice issues, build knowledge for the future, and use that knowledge to prepare new and advanced practitioners.

Roy's lifelong mission of defining nursing for clinical practice began in 1964 as a master's student, specializing in Pediatric Nursing, at the University of California at Los Angeles. The discussion topic of the first seminar in an advanced Pediatric class was to articulate *the goal of nursing*. Roy described it as *promoting patient adaptation*. Her clinical experience in pediatric nursing had provided insights into the resilence of children and their families in managing changing health concerns. The nurse's role, then, seemed to be enhancing this natural process in every way possible in all areas of practice. From this insight, with the encouragement of Dorothy Johnson, came the nearly thirty years of fruitful work deriving the basic elements of the model and constantly interrelating the theoretical elements with Roy's own practice and research and that of countless colleagues around the world.

The first publication on the Roy Adaptation Model appeared in the nursing literature in 1970 (Roy, 1970). The model has evolved through the years with significant growth in its use for nursing education particularly in the 1970s, for nursing practice in the 1980s, and greater research in the 1990s. Evidence of this growth lies in such facts as: graduates of programs with Roy Model based curricula by 1985 were estimated at several hundred thousand (Andrews, 1987). These graduates and a new wave of clinically committed nurses with graduate degrees are making a difference in model-based practice. Although complete literature reviews are difficult to obtain (see Johnson, 1989), one recent survey located 210 articles on the Roy Adaptation Model (Barone & Roy, 1992). The majority of these related to use of the model in nursing practice. However, 64 citations were research-based. The analysis and synthesis of the extant literature for clinical nursing science is a current project of a recently founded core group of scholars working on the model's basic and clinical sciences (Pollock, et al. in review).

ESSENTIALS OF THE MODEL

Nursing's goal is to contribute to the overall goal of health care, that is, promoting the health of individuals and society. More specifically, according to the Roy Adaptation Model, nursing acts to enhance the interaction of the person with the environment to promote adaptation. Promoting adaptation in the four modes identified by Roy contributes to the patient's health and quality of life.

Understanding the major concepts of the model is based on a review of the scientific and philosophic assumptions of the Roy Adaptation Model (Roy, 1988a; Roy & Andrews, 1991). The scientific assumptions are associated with von Bertalanffy's (1968) General Systems Theory, and Helson's (1964) Adaptation-Level Theory. The assumptions from *systems theory* include:

- Holism - a system is a set of units so related or connected as to form a unity or whole.

- Interdependence - a system is a whole that functions as a whole by virtue of the interdependence of its parts.

- Control Processes - a system has inputs, outputs, and control and feedback processes.

- Information Feedback - input, in the form of a standard or feedback, often is referred to as information, and

- Complexity of Living Systems - living systems are almost infinitely more complex than mechanical systems and have standards and feedback to direct their functioning as a whole.

Additionally, assumptions from *adaptation-level theory* are as follows:

- Behavior as Adaptive - human behavior represents adaptation to environmental and organismic forces.

- Adaptation as a Function of Stimuli and Adaptation Level-adaptive behavior is a function of the stimulus and adaptation level, that is, the pooled effect of the focal, contextual, and residual stimuli.

- Individual, Dynamic Adaptation Levels - adaptation is a process of responding positively to environmental changes; this positive response decreases the responses necessary to cope with the stimuli and increases sensitivity to respond to other stimuli, and

- Positive and Active Processes of Responding - responses reflect the state of the organism as well as the properties of stimuli and hence are regarded as active processes.

These assumptions established Roy's belief in holism and in the person as the initiator of adaptive processes. The patterning of these processes in exchange with the environment allows one's adaptive abilities to provide the dynamic energy for health and effective living.

Principles of humanism and veritivity are the source for the philosophical assumptions of the model. *Humanism* assumes:

- Creativity - person's own creative power.

- Purposefulness - person's behavior is purposeful and not merely a chain of cause and effect.

- Holism - person is holistic, and

- Interpersonal process - the interpersonal relationship is significant.

The principle of *veritivity* is partially based on the Teilhardian (de Chardin, 1959; de Chardin, 1965) view of the universe and the orthogenesis of humankind. It enlightens the model with the following assumptions:

- Purposefulness of human existence,

- Unity of purpose,

- Activity, creativity, and

- Value and meaning of life.

These philosophical assumptions stem from Roy's lifelong study, conviction, and living of a theologically-based religious faith. In addition Roy built upon both undergraduate and graduate studies in philosophy, especially related to the nature of person and the place of persons in a cosmos set in motion by a loving Creator. Early on she studied the philosophies of Aristotle and Thomas Aquinas, as well as the philosophical roots and historical methods of hermeneutical exegesis of biblical texts. Later the works of Freud, Jung, Adler, de Chardin, Kant, Hegel, Marx and Freire were added. A strong basis in sociology, social psychology, and anthropology opened doors into structural analysis, empirical deductive knowledge strategies, interactionist theory, and phenomenology. Current teaching of the epistemology of nursing has allowed Roy to study the philosophy of science movements affecting nursing over the past few decades and the thinking of current nurse philosophers.

The assumptions identified here provide the scientific foundation of the Roy Adaptation Model, and direct the values and beliefs to be included in defining metaparadigmatic concepts of person, health, environment, and nursing. Each concept will he described briefly and the derivation of these concepts from the basic assumptions will be noted.

THE ADAPTIVE PERSON/ GROUP

The person is the focus of nursing and in the Roy Adaptation Model the key concept is person as adaptive system. Theoretical frameworks representing persons as adaptive systems have been developed on the individual level (Roy & McLeod, 1981) and for persons in groups in society, such as family (Roy, 1983), community (Hanchett, 1988), and organizational groups (Roy & Anway, 1989; Lutjens, 1990). Internal processes for coping on the individual level have been termed the regulator and the cognator. For the organizational group they are categorized as stabilizer and innovator. The focus of this discussion is on the person as an individual.

Early in the development of the model, content analysis of 500 samples of patient behavior in all areas of clinical practice revealed four facets of the individual's adaptive status: physiologic, self concept, role function, and interdependence. The adaptive modes reflect the adaptive processes and can be the foci for nursing assessments and the variables for research. Roy has used the analogy of the kaleidoscope as an image of the holistic interrelatedness of the adaptive modes and of how the modes change in fluid ways to manifest the patterns of the human situation. The inner dynamism of cognator/regulator processes generates these patterns in a holistic way, based on the scientific and philosophical assumptions of the model.

The person is seen as part of organismic forces with the propensity for self-determining fulfillment of the purposefulness of human existence. The cognitive-emotional processes of the cognator act within varying levels of consciousness as the person deals with internal and external states. The neuro-chemical-endocrine processes of the regulator may be outside of consciousness, but provide the substrates of human conscious processes and action. Nurses are becoming involved in the developing field of psychoneuroendocrinology because of what it can tell them about the possibilities for human behavior, as well as interventions to promote and measure individual adaptive processes. Behaviors can be described as adaptive or ineffective on the basis of whether or not they promote integrity by meeting the goals of adaptation, that is, survival, growth, reproduction, and mastery.

ENVIRONMENT

The environment contains input to the person or group, and includes internal and external stimuli. Derived from the scientific assumptions of Helson's (1964) adaptation level theory, the stimuli are categorized as focal, contextual, and residual. The cognator and regulator systems interface in an organismic way with the internal and external stimuli. Roy found Helson's categories of stimuli useful within the adaptation framework. First, focal stimuli are described as that most immediate to a person and can be internal and/or external stimuli. Secondly, contextual stimuli refers to all other stimuli present in the situation. Lastly, residual stimuli are part of the person's interaction with the environment as the total cosmos, both elements within the person's awareness and those that are not, but are not as easily analyzed as part of the current person-environment interaction. More broadly, environmental stimuli include all the conditions, circumstances, and influences surrounding, and affecting the development and behavior of the person or group.

Significant stimuli in all human adaptation include stage of development, family, and culture. The use of the term stimuli sometimes has been misinterpreted as related to the framework of behaviorism. The language of behaviorism was in wide use during early stages of the Roy model development, however, it was clear from the beginning that Roy used the classes of stimuli to describe the complexity of the environment taken in by the person, and never referred to stimulus-response effects. In fact, each category of stimuli is highly relevant to the established model assumptions.

The multiple inputs, outputs, and dynamism of forming adaptation levels is compatible with organismic systems theory. Focal stimuli are another way to identify the patient's felt need, as identified by other nurse writers. Roy's emphasis on context pre-dates the current burgeoning literature in this area. Given the humanistic assumptions of the model, and the value of the person within a common human destiny, the adaptation nursing model nurse is interested in the intra and interpersonal contextual factors as well as specific empirics of the setting. The category of residual stimuli is particularly compatible with the philosophical assumptions about the person. In Helson's physiological psychology experiments, he always found that equations of human responses were off from his predictions by a certain x factor, which he called the residuals, to account for the factors within the person that had not been specified in his empirical work. Roy puts this notion together with her beliefs about the person and finds that residual stimuli may be those which the nurse has not yet assessed or of which the nurse and/or the person is not aware for whatever reason. In addition, always being aware of a category for residual stimuli allows for the mystery in each person since each is unique within the common destiny and the nurse may not expect to know the other as the other knows self or is known by the Creator.

Adaptive responses are a function of the stimulus, or environmental change, and the adaptation level of the person or group (Helson, 1964). Further, adaptation level is described as a changing point that represents the person's ability to respond positively in a situation.

HEALTH

Nursing's goal is to promote adaptation and thereby contribute to health. According to the Roy Adaptation Model, health is a state and a process of being and becoming an integrated and whole person. Integrity implies soundness or an unimpaired condition that can lead to completeness or unity. Adaptation, then, is a process of promoting integrity, or one may also say that adaptation means interacting positively with the environment and thereby promoting health. One's health does not depend on the absence or presence of disease, rather it relates to use of the processes that lead to patterns of integrity of the person and the ability to move toward effective unity of the adaptive modes. Roy has addressed the issue raised by critics as to whether adaptation is a process and health is a product. It is more in keeping with the assumptions of the model and with the concept of adaptation developed by Roy (Roy & Roberts, 1981; Roy, 1990, and Roy & Andrews, 1991) that both are viewed as on-going processes. Basically, a process is a series of states; a process is a series of actions toward an end. On the other hand, a state is the condition relative to the environment. In nursing assessment or in clinical research, it may be appropriate to look at adaptation or health as an outcome of the on-going processes, and thus as a state for that point in time, but the clinical assessment and research on the processes of adaptation and of health are primary.

ADAPTATION NURSING

According to this theoretical model, nursing is defined as the science and the practice of promoting adaptation for individuals and groups in situations involving health and illness. Nursing assessment focuses specifically on the person's adaptive and ineffective behavior and the stimuli or factors influencing it. The model views nursing diagnosis in any one of three ways: statement of behaviors and stimuli that are the focus; summary label within an adaptive mode; or label to summarize a behavioral pattern with more than one mode being affected by the same stimuli. Nursing goals or standards are stated as adaptive behaviors expected as an outcome of nursing intervention. Given the uniqueness and value of each individual, highlighted in the assumptions, it is clear that each of these steps is handled within the nurse/patient relationship with the person being the source of adaptive processes. Nursing interventions are planned to help manage stimuli that promote adaptive processes. Finally, the nurse is involved with the person in evaluation or reassessment to determine whether or not the person's goal of adaptive behavior was reached.

Nursing practice is based upon the clinical science of nursing. Two substantive areas of clinical knowledge in this model are the cognator and regulator processes and the four adaptive modes. Roy identified these knowledge components in early work and has amplified and clarified them through the years, at times in significant collaboration with others. The research focus on both cognator/regulator processes and adaptive modes intensifies as a way to bring the theory to practice.

KNOWLEDGE FOR PRACTICE

Roy (Roy, 1991a) derived a structure of knowledge based on the Roy Adaptation Model. Nursing is divided into two sciences, the basic nursing science and a clinical nursing science. The basic science of nursing focuses on understanding the person and health as defined by the model. Topics include: adaptive processes such as cognator-regulator activity; stabilizer-innovator activity; stability of adaptive patterns; and dynamics of evolving adaptive patterns. The basic science of the adaptive modes includes their development, interrelatedness, and cultural and other influences. Person and environment interaction and integration of adaptive modes are investigated to add to the basic science of adaptation related to health.

The relationship of theory to practice is the mandate of all theoretical work in a practice discipline. Roy notes (1991b) that nursing practice in the next century will be differentiated by the needs of practice and by the knowledge created to meet those needs. The model provides a framework and language to describe health care practice needs, both for individuals and society. The central theme of the clinical science based on the Roy Adaptation Model is enhancing patient adaptation. Substantive basic nursing knowledge is called upon in this effort. In clinical studies one looks at changes in cognator-regulator and stabilizer-innovator effectiveness, changes within and among the adaptive modes and nursing care to promote adaptive processes. The nurse can look at the overall effectiveness of adaptive processes, for example, looking at a cognator process such as motor response sequencing, and can help the person evaluate how effective the pattern of activity is in meeting his or her goals.

Cognator/Regulator Processes. Roy conceptualized an adaptive system's control process as originating from an internal control mechanism. The mechanism contains processes that are both innate and acquired. In turn, the cognator and regulator subsystems are defined as types of adaptive processes. Roy's early work (Roy, 1970) listed the cognator subsystem as responding via: (a) perceptual and information processing, (b) learning, (c) judging, and (d) emotion. In contrast, the regulator subsystem responds automatically via: (a) neural, (b) chemical, and (c) endocrine processes.

The further theoretical articulation of these mechaisms has been carried out in stages through the years using qualitative research, conceptual derivation and quantitative research. From the earliest work, cognitive/emotional and regulatory mechanisms were defined and described as channels by which persons adapt and reach higher levels of wellness. The question pursued has been to identify the characteristics and components of cognator/regulator processes and how these are used by individuals in different situations. The underlying theoretical base derives from the cognator subsystem of the Roy model (Roy & McLeod, 1981), a nursing model for cognitive processing (Roy, 1988b), and the Das/Luria model of simultaneous and successive information processing (Das, Kirby, Jarman, 1979). The empirical base was developed from two qualitative interview studies, content analysis of nursing process care plans (Roy, 1975), as well as clinical research in patient information processing which Roy conducted from 1983–1988.

From the qualitative studies of patient interviews and nursing process content analysis, Roy identified 45 categories of cognator coping reflecting the adaptation in the psychosocial modes. For example, for the person in the hospital, a frequent cognitive strategy when one is unable to respond to usual demands is selective attention. That is, people shut out other demands and focus on those useful to them for getting well and promoting health. Later, Roy developed the nursing model of cognitive processing (Roy, 1988b). The broad domains of cognitive processing lie in five categories: input, central, and output processes, activity and emotion. These in turn contain 11 major processes, such as arousal and attention, which are further analyzed into 27 cognitive processes available for interaction with the environment. For example, arousal and attention can be examined further by looking at selective attention, speed of processing, and alertness.

These two typologies were synthesized by Roy in 1992 (Roy, in progress) and a survey instrument to measure cognitve adaptation processing was derived. Simultaneously empirical studies using the original four cognator categories in an 11-item instrument were completed (Frederickson & Roy, in progress). Based on the theoretical and empirical development, and the promising findings of the first 11-item instrument, Roy set about the development and, with colleagues, testing of the survey instrument that might confirm or further clarify the dimensions of the cognator. This testing can then provide a valid and reliable measure of positive cognator processing. The first extended 72-item version of the tool is the Cognitive Adaptation Processing Scale (CAPS) and a 49-item version, tapping the same cognitive domains, has been developed for use with elders. Several cohorts of data will be analyzed to report the outcome of this work. Another of Roy's colleagues (Hassey-Dow, 1992) has developed a scale looking at cognator adaptive processes in cancer patients. This scale has excellent psychometric properties and already is in demand for research in the field. Much more remains to be known about cognator processing, but it is already clear that this work, based on the model's assumptions about persons, offers a view of adaptation and coping that differs from that in the literature of either the biological or the social sciences.

Another major area of on-going theoretical and empirical research relates to the regulator mechanism and the interrelatedness of cognator and regulator processes. Advances in the field of neuroendocrinology can provide both insights and data as to the nature and function of these processes.

Adaptive Modes. The cognator and regulator adaptive subsystems respond to various stimuli and these responses are manifested in human behavior that reflects the person. As noted above, the categories of adaptive modes, or behavioral ways of adapting, that are developed for use in clinical practice and are studied in nursing science include: (a) the physiological mode, (b) the self concept mode, (c) the role function mode, and (d) the interdependence mode.

The physiological mode contains physical coping mechanisms to promote a system's integrity. For example, oxygenation, nutrition, elimination, activity/rest, and protection are recognized as basic needs of a person as adaptive system, and proper functioning of the senses, fluids/electrolytes, neurologic, and endocrine activities are also needed for physiological integrity. The innate and acquired mechanisms for meeting such needs and proper functioning manifest themselves in this mode. Clinical knowledge includes the stable and effective processes for each under usual or altered conditions.

The self concept mode focuses on spiritual and psychological coping mechanisms to promote a system's integrity. Driever (1976a & b) described the self concept within the nursing model as including a personal self and physical self. Some key characteristics of the personal self are self consistency, self ideal, and moral ethical self. These characteristics form the core beliefs at the center of ones being about who one is. This core self, then, greatly influences ones behavior. Within a topology of indicators of positive adaptation (Roy & Andrews, 1991), for the personal self the nurse assesses a stable pattern of self consistency, effective integration of self-ideal, effective processes of moral-ethical-spiritual growth, functional self esteem and effective coping strategies for threats to self. Thus, nurses using the model are directed to be aware of knowledge development related to the adaptation of the self, such as empowerment, hope, and transcendence.

The role function mode (Malaznik, 1976; Randell, 1976) promotes a system's social integrity by defining the individual in relation to others. People have primary roles based on age and social situation. One is an active participant in creating and carrying out roles by way of instrumental, goal-oriented, and expressive, emotion-based, behaviors. Secondary and tertiary roles accompany one's primary roles and provide for auxiliary social functions. For example, a woman may have a career in nursing or medicine, but adopt a child and thus take on secondary roles of parenting such as taking a turn as home-room mother at the child's school.

Clinical knowledge about the role function mode focuses on such topics as effective processes of role transition, integration of instrumental and expressive roles, stable patterns of role mastery, and effective processes for coping with role changes. Much literature is now available on gender role development and functioning that is highly relevant to clinical knowledge in nursing.

Finally, the interdependence mode reflects the person's integrity by providing affectional adequacy through significant others and support systems (Tedrow, 1984). Receptive and contributive behavior are identified as key behaviors inherent in the interdependence mode. One gives and receives love, value, and respect within this mode. In addition to enhancing the person's receptive and contributive behaviors, the nurse also acts within the interdependence mode with patients. Current conceptual and empirical work on nursing as a science of caring is relevant here. The typology of indicators of positive adaptation (Roy & Andrews, 1991) lists the following foci for clinical knowledge: stable pattern of giving and receiving nurturing; affectional adequacy; effective pattern of aloneness and relating; and effective coping strategies for separation and loneliness.

These four adaptive modes and their indicators of positive adaptation, and the related recurring adaptation problems identified within the model (Roy & Andrews, 1991) serve as a guide to assess a person's responses, consequently, assessing adaptation level. Responses that promote integrity in terms of the goals of the human system are termed adaptive responses. Nursing knowledge for practice is derived from the understanding of the modes and how the cognator and regulator act to promote adaptation and the unity of the modes. This effective cognator/regulator activity which integrates the total person is known as health.

FUTURE DIRECTIONS

The structure of knowledge that Roy has outlined provides both knowledge for practice and direction for future knowledge development. The basic content and process of the model have been identified (Andrews & Roy, 1986) for nurses to apply and participate in. Much work can be done by nurse scholars in practice as well as academia to continue the clarification and expansion of the model. Basing a structure of knowledge on patterns and processes allows for the expansion of that structure for the development of new knowledge to meet the changing needs of practice (Roy, 1991b). For example, multiple organ transplants and artificial organs raise questions about how nurses may assist the person in this situation to maintain a stable pattern of self-consistency. How will we maintain the value of the human person when we enter the post-indiscriminate technologic era? These questions relate both to the adaptive processes of the individual and of social groups.

Within the developing understanding of cognator/regulator processes and the adaptive modes lies the challenge to identify nursing interventions that can best enhance adaptation and health for the person. Similar challenges present themselves when dealing with families, communities, and other social structures as adaptive systems. The Roy Adaptation Model provides an instrument for the task before the profession in moving into the next century. A clear vision of nursing can provide a centering point for dealing with the issues of our post-modern information-processing world. Nursing can create the change that promotes personal life fulfillment and a new social order.

REFERENCES

Andrews, H. A. (1987). *Curricular implementation of the Roy adaptation model.* Doctoral dissertation, University of Alberta, Edmonton.

Andrews, H. A., and Roy, C. (1986). *Essentials of the Roy adaptation model.* Norwalk, CT: Appleton-Century-Crofts.

Barone, S. H., and Roy, C. (1992, April). *Instruments used in research with the Roy adaptation model: A synthesis of the literature.* Paper presented at the meeting of the Eastern Nursing Research Society, Washington, DC.

Das, J. P., Kirby, J. R., and Jarman, R. F. (1979). *Simultaneous and successive cognitive processes.* New York: Academic Press.

de Chardin, P. T. (1959). *The phenomenon of man.* New York: Harper & Row.

de Chardin, P. T. (1965). *Hymn of the universe* (S. Bartholomew, Trans.). New York: Harper & Row.

Driever, M. J. (1976a). Development of self-concept. In C. Roy, *Introduction to nursing: An adaptation model* (pp. 180–191). Englewood Cliffs, NJ: Prentice-Hall, Inc.

Driever, M. J. (1976b). Theory of self-concept. In C. Roy, *Introduction to nursing: An adaptation model* (pp. 169–179) Englewood Cliffs, NJ: Prentice-Hall, Inc.

Frederickson, K. and C. Roy. (in preparation). *Cognator effectiveness in a study of lives of professionals.*

Hanchett, E. S. (1988). *Nursing frameworks and community as client: Bridging the gap.* Norwalk, CT: Appleton & Lange.

Hassey-Dow, K. (1992). *Surviving and having children after the breast cancer experience.* Doctoral dissertation, Boston College, Boston.

Helson, H. (1964). *Adaptation level theory.* NY: Harper & Row.

Johnson, E. D. (1989). In search of application of nursing theories: The nursing citation index. *Bulletin, Medical Librarians Association.* 72(2), 176–184.

Lutjens, L. R. (1990). Relationships between medical condition, nursing condition, nursing intensity, medical severity and length of stay in hospitalized medical-surgical adults using the theory of social organizations as adaptive systems. (Doctoral dissertation, Wayne State University) *Dissertation Abstracts International, 52,* 03B.

Malaznik, N. (1976). Theory of role function. In C. Roy, *Introduction to nursing: An adaptation model.* Englewood Cliffs, NJ: Prentice-Hall, Inc.

Pollack, S., Fredrickson, K., Carson, M., Massey, V., and Roy, C. (in review). State of the science: Deriving middle-range theories for clinical practice from model-based research. *Image, Journal of Nursing Scholarship.*

Randell, B. (1976). Development of role function. In C. Roy, *Introduction to nursing: An adaptation model.* Englewood Cliffs, NJ: Prentice-Hall, Inc.

Roy, C. (1970). Adaptation: A conceptual framework for nursing, *Nursing Outlook,* 18(3), 43–45.

Roy, C. (1975). *Psycho-social adaptation and the coping mechanisms.* Unpublished paper, Clinical site, Queen of the Valley Hospital, West Covina, CA.

Roy, C. (1983). Roy adaptation model and analysis and application to the expectant family and the family in primary care. In L. Clements & F. B. Roberts, *Family health: A theoretical approach to nursing care* (pp. 255–278, 298–303; and 375–378). NY: John Wiley and Sons.

Roy, C. (1988a). An explication of the philosophical assumptions of the Roy adaptation model. *Nursing Science Quarterly*, l(l), 26–34.

Roy, C. (1988b). Alterations in cognitive processing. In P. Mitchel, L. Hodges, M. Muwaswes, and C. Walleck. (Eds.). *American Association of Neuroscience Nurses: Phenomena and Practice*. (pp. 185–211). Norwalk, CT: Appleton & Lange.

Roy, C. (1990). Theorist's response to "Strengthening the Roy adaptation model through conceptual clarification." *Nursing Science Quarterly*, 3(2), 64–66.

Roy, C. (1991a). The Roy adaptation model in nursing research. In C. Roy and H. Andrews, *The Roy adaptation model: The definitive statement*. (pp. 445–458). Norwalk, CT: Appleton & Lange.

Roy, C. (1991b). Structure of knowledge: Paradigm, model and research specifications for differential practice. In American Academy of Nursing Proceedings of 18th annual meeting *Differentiating Nursing Practice into the twenty-first century* (pp. 31–40). Kansas City, MO: American Academy of Nursing.

Roy, C. (in preparation). *Cognitive adaptation processing scale (CAPS): Derivation and testing*.

Roy, C., & Andrews, H. (1991). *The Roy adaptation model: The definitive statement*. Norwalk, CT: Appleton & Lange.

Roy, C., & Anway, J. (1989). Roy's adaptation model: Theories and propositions for administration. In H. B. DiVincenti, C. Arndt, and J. Marriner, *Dimensions and issues in administration*. St. Louis: Mosby.

Roy, C., & McLeod, D. (1981). Theory of the person as an adaptive system. In C. Roy, and S. Roberts, *Theory construction in nursing: An adaptation model* (pp. 49–69). Englewood Cliffs, NJ: Prentice Hall.

Roy, C., & Roberts, S. (1981). *Theory construction in nursing: An adaptation model*. Englewood Cliffs, NJ: Prentice Hall.

Tedrow, M. P. (1984). Interdependence: Theory and development. In C. Roy, *Introduction to nursing: An adaptation model* (2nd ed.). Englewood Cliffs, NJ: Prentice-Hall, Inc.

von Bertalanffy, L. (1968). *General systems theory*. NY: Braziller.

16

Translating the Roy Adaptation Model into Practice and Research

Keville Frederickson

INTRODUCTION

For the last five years, I have been working with the Roy Adaptation Model (RAM) in nursing practice, research and education. The model has served as the organizing framework for all my nursing activities. Using one model for clinical practice, education, and research promoted a logical foundation for building nursing knowledge. It also provided an opportunity to demonstrate the versatility and the practicality of nursing models, specifically the Roy Adaptation Model.

One outcome has been a program of research focusing on adaptation among a variety of patients including those with cancer, AIDS, and neurosurgical and cardiac diagnoses.

Another result, the focus of this chapter, has been the development of a clinical nursing unit which applied the RAM to nursing practice. This unit has been featured in a videotape highlighting the implementation of the model for education and clinlcal practice (*Excellence in Action*, 1991).

DISSONANCE BETWEEN THEORY AND PRACTICE

My interest in conceptual models began when I was the director of a graduate nursing program, responsible for teaching the graduate course on nursing theory. After teaching the course a number of times I experienced a lack of credibility. There were no opportunities locally for students to observe the translation of theory into practice. I was unable to continue teaching a course that seemed to have little observable practical application and maintain my teaching credibility.

In response to this dissonance between theory and practice, I developed a proposal for operationalizing a nursing model in a clinical setting. The proposal included a pilot whereby I rolled up my sleeves and after 20 years of being away from the bedside, provided direct patient care with the staff nurses for three months. I was fortunate to have a wonderful preceptor and at the end of the pilot it became clear that this staff and unit were ideal for the total project. I also realized that staff nursing is not for the weak or the fainthearted. To facilitate the project, a joint appointment was arranged between the college where I was teaching and a major medical center. The goal of the joint appointment was to establish a theory-based unit that would be a center for clinical practice.

ASSUMPTIONS UNDERLYING THEORY-BASED PRACTICE

The project was based on two assumptions about professional nursing practice: 1) that professional nursing practice is autonomous nursing practice, which means that nursing controls its own practice, and 2) that autonomous professional nursing practice cannot exist unless it is based on a nursing conceptual system (Frederickson, 1991).

I believe that autonomous professional nursing practice must be based on a nursing conceptual model. Following this project, I am now more convinced than ever that autonomous nursing practice requires a foundation that can only be provided through a nursing theory framework.

Nursing models provide a basis for independent decisions that preclude permission from other disciplines. In a hospital setting, interventions are more likely to parallel those of medicine when nursing care is based on the medical diagnosis. Nursing frequently requests permission for innovative interventions when practice uses a medical orientation rather than a nursing model.

Nursing's contributions are collaborative as well as integrative when care is based on a nursing model. For example, discharge planning based on the modes of the RAM may be directed toward maintaining a level of physical functioning (physiological mode), enhancing self esteem (self concept mode), returning the patient to prior roles (role function mode), and enlisting the support of significant others in the planning (interdependence mode). Each of these goals combines the expertise of other disciplines but requires the integration provided by the RAM to formulate a plan that illustrates the uniqueness of nursing.

The application of a nursing model has the potential to enhance the nurse's self esteem especially in the doctor/nurse relationship. Through observations, when nurses practice from a more medical perspective they compete with the physician for supremacy of medical knowledge primarily in the area of pathophysiology. Since nurses have not received a medical education, eventually their contributions can only be less than and/or inferior to the physician's. Consequently the nurse feels less self confident. By using a model designed for nursing, which views the patient as a whole, the nurse has an opportunity for distinct contributions to patient care. These nursing contributions are then different from those of medicine and recognize the nurse's superiority within the domain of nursing knowledge.

Collaboration between nursing and medicine is more likely to be based on mutual respect when each is based on its own distinct body of knowledge. For example, in our Neurosurgical ICU, nursing's emphasis had been on the physiological components of patient care. Therefore, the dimensions nurses and physicians addressed were similar, such as neurosurgical signs, neuropathophysiology and indicated neurosurgical procedures. Since implementing the nursing model more emphasis has been placed on the integration of the psychosocial needs of the patient with the physiological. It is this integration that served to differentiate a nursing focus from one that is medical. With the new emphasis, nursing addressed the interplay between the physiological and psychosocial components of the person such as the effects of visitors on intercranial pressure and vital signs.

SELECTION OF THE ROY ADAPTATION MODEL

In selecting a nursing model, my preference was for one that viewed the person as an integrated whole yet recognized the many parts and clearly addressed the physiological component as one of these parts. This type of nursing model was needed in an acute care setting to enhance communication between medicine and nursing. A framework for patient care was needed that allowed us to find a common ground yet one that promoted nursing's uniqueness.

The RAM (Roy & Andrews, 1991) sees the person as a biopsychosocial whole which served as a much needed link for the project. Discussions with physicians about the basis for my practice turned out to be relatively easy. In fact, one neurosurgeon boasted following my case presentation at Neurosurgical rounds, that he considers the same things I do, only not in such an organized manner.

THE PURPOSE OF THE PROJECT

The purpose of the project was to increase the autonomy of the registered nurse's practice through theory-based practice. A related goal of the project was to develop and evaluate strategies that would improve autonomy and likewise, enhance retention and recruitment.

Attracting and keeping qualified nurses was a real problem for this unit. There was a high turnover and high vacancy rates. Much of the research on retention and recruitment such as the Magnet Study (American Academy of Nursing, 1983) and the reports from the National Commission on Nursing (1981) indicated that autonomy or control over practice, as well as control over personal time, contributes to nurse satisfaction. It seemed that the introduction of a nursing model as a vehicle for autonomy would enhance recruitment and retention.

Another goal of the project was to initiate a relationship between nursing service and nursing practice that would be advantageous for both. Nursing service needs the research findings and theoretical bases that education can provide and education needs the reality-orientation that service can offer.

TRANSLATING THEORY INTO PRACTICE: THE DEVELOPMENT OF A ROLE

My position, clinical nurse scientist, was viewed as an important role to develop. As an educator, it was my responsibility to provide the leadership for the interpretation and translation of nursing science research and theory into practice.

Over these past four years I have found that it is not easy to apply a nursing model to practice. It requires in-depth knowledge of the model, repeated applications to a wide range of patient care situations, synthesizing the evaluations of the model's usefulness with patients, continual discussions with practicing nurses and nurse theoreticians, application of the revisions at the bedside and finally, development of educational materials for teaching the application of the model.

IMPLEMENTING THE MODEL

The implementation of theory-based practice utilized the RAM as the framework for change. Therefore, facilitators of the change, myself and the unit-based project director, directed the education of the staff toward either enhancing the control processes or developing coping skills. These two approaches are utilized as interventions according to the RAM. Also consistent with the RAM was the goal of assisting nurses to incorporate the new approach to patient care (the stimulus) or adapt the environment so that conceptually-based practice was part of it (Frederickson, 1991). For example, the work environment was modified to allow time and support for using the nursing model. We introduced a nursing care conference which viewed patient case studies from the Roy Adaptation perspective; an assessment form was developed which utilized the nursing model. The nurses adaptation skills were enhanced by providing time away from the unit to plan the assessment forms; by providing rewards in the system such as pictures that were featured in a regional newsletter, displays in the hospital lobby, membership on special committees and/or cameo appearances in a national videotape for those who championed the utilization of the model.

We used a variety of environmental stimuli to present and reinforce the model. The intention was to keep the idea of the RAM for practice on everyone's mind. We developed materials and forums for incorporating the RAM such as including the RAM in the unit-based orientation. In addition, nursing/medical rounds, I occasionally presented a patient case to the nurses and neurosurgical residents using the RAM.

The nursing care conference always utilized the RAM format to present nursing cases. Frequently the emphasis of the case presented was on understanding and applying the model for nursing care.

The unit-based director of the project initiated a number of innovations, such as a bulletin board display presenting a case study using the model. In addition, a nursing model journal club was formed and a self-learning module was developed. Potential candidates for nursing positions were asked about their comfort in using the Roy model for practice.

RESULTS OF THE EVALUATION

A study was designed to evaluate the effectiveness of the project using a control unit for comparison. The control unit was matched for bed-size (approximately 38 beds), acuity level, nurse-patient ratio (approximately 4:1), and the presence of an ICU on the unit. All nurses on both units were invited to participate and were tested at baseline and then 18 months later.

Briefly, the study design included a number of standardized instruments as well as additional data on nurse satisfaction, such as pursuit of education and retention and recruitment of nurses on each unit. The details of this study are reported elsewhere (Frederickson, 1991). The variables identified were nurses' perception of their work environment, self esteem, collaborative practice, work satisfaction and patient satisfaction.

The results were based on 28 nurses from the experimental or theory-based practice unit and 26 nurses from the control unit. In general there was no difference in collaborative practice between the two units at baseline or over time. The nurses on the experimental unit reported a significant increase in satisfaction with cohesion, control, potential for innovation, and general comfort as well as an improved sense of professional status. Self esteem also increased significantly on the unit using the RAM as compared to the control unit. Patients reported more satisfaction on the experimental unit, however, the level did not reach significance. Additionally 42 percent of the 47 full-time nurses on the theory-based practice unit returned to school for further education.

Retention improved on the experimental unit. During the first year, ten nurses left the experimental unit as compared to no resignations during the next year. The control unit traditionally had a very high retention rate which did not change during the course of the study. The replacement of one nurse on the Neurosurgical unit cost about $30,000. By retaining ten nurses, the institution saved about $300,000 during that one year.

Qualitative data included observations and discussions with the nursing staff. A few nurses shared that they approached patients differently after using the RAM. As one nurse commented, "I feel very drawn to the patients using the Roy model—it is no longer the glioblastoma in 320 but the 40-year old woman with three young children struggling to adapt to feelings of mortality."

Families also reported being treated differently on this unit. As one family stated, "We feel that we are 'the patient.' We're always included in the things the nurse does for our mother as part of the nurse's concern."

SUMMARY

The use of one lens for viewing nursing has been a valuable asset in the development of nursing knowledge. Research and the conceptual development of interventions utilizing one model have produced the foundation for a program of nursing research and nursing practice (Strauman, Frederickson, & Jackson, 1987; Jackson, Strauman, Frederickson, & Strauman, 1991; Frederickson, Jackson, Strauman, & Strauman, 1991; Frederickson, 1991; Frederickson, 1992; Frederickson, 1993).

The implementation of the RAM as a basis for nursing practice was the result of a personal need to create a place where nursing students could observe the implementation of a nursing model. One unit was developed as a pilot. The results appeared very promising with significant improvements in nurses' perceptions of self, their work environment and retention. The pilot unit was successful. Although administration was supportive of the RAM, the culture of the remainder of the institution was not prepared for the introduction and utilization of the model. Currently, there is a major initiative to create a culture that will support institutional changes (Jackson, Filippino, Frederickson, Brennan, & Akan, 1992). Whether the institution adopts the RAM or another nursing model as the basis for their practice is unclear at this time.

What I learned from this project was that a nursing model could be established and provide a sense of pride in the nurses about their practice. The use of a nursing model was an attraction that recruited new nurses, student nurses and graduate nurses as observers. Translating nursing theory into daily practice is possible but requires bonding between nurse theorists, nurse educators, and nurse clinicians. This project did provide a link between nursing service and nursing education and medicine, each understanding the other better as we worked together to improve the condition of the patient.

Most importantly for me, this experience was a daily reminder of why I chose nursing as a career—to be with people in distress and provide comfort through patient care. This project allowed me to synthesize all that I had learned in nursing and utilize it in direct patient care, teaching and research, with the guidance and support of colleagues and mentors.

ACKNOWLEDGMENTS

The opportunity to develop a theory-based nursing unit was stimulated through an idea planted by Dr. Rosanne Wille, then Dean of Nursing at Lehman College, allowed to grow and facilitated by Elaine Brennan, Director of Nursing at Montefiore Medical Center, Moses Division and continuously nurtured by Sr. Callista Roy. Although everyone on the Neurosurgical unit assisted in the development of the practice unit, a few were particularly instrumental such as, Debra Hanna, the unit-based project director and Brigette Niesen, the Administrative Supervisor. The support from the Chief of Neurosurgery, Dr. Paul Kornblith, enhanced the communication between medicine and nursing and provided an unusual boost for nursing models. The nurses on the unit all worked very hard to understand and apply a new way of viewing patients. Particular gratitude is owed to the patients and their families who displayed continuous heroism as they dealt with devastating conditions. Their adaptations will remain a source of inspiration for me forever.

REFERENCES

American Academy of Nursing (1983). *Magnet hospitals: Attraction and retention of professional nurses.* Kansas City, MO: American Nurses Association.

Excellence in Action: *Application of the Roy adaptation model* (1992). St. Louis: CV Mosby.

Frederickson, K., Jackson, B., Strauman, T., & Strauman, J. (1991).

Testing hypotheses derived from the Roy adaptation model. *Nursing Science Quarterly*, 4:168–174.

Frederickson, K. (1991). Application of the Roy Adaptation Model: Basis for differentiating practice. In American Academy of Nursing's *Proceedings of Annual Meeting Differentiating Nursing Practice: Into the Twenty-First Century*, 41–44.

Frederickson, K. (1992). Research methodology and nursing science. *Nursing Science Quarterly*, 5(4):150–151.

Frederickson, K. (1993). Using a nursing model to manage symptoms: Anxiety and the Roy adaptation model. *Holistic Nursing Practice*, 7(2):36–42.

Jackson, B., Strauman, J., Frederickson, K., & Strauman, T. (1991). Long-term biopsychosocial effects of Interleukin-2 therapy. *Oncology Nursing Forum*, 18:683–690.

Jackson, B., Filippino, J., Frederickson, K., Brennan, E., & Akan, A. (1992). Cultural change in a complex nursing service. *Nursing Dynamics*, 1(2):14–19.

National Commission on Nursing (1981). *Initial report and preliminary recommendations*. Chicago: The Hospital Research and Educational Trust.

Roy, C., & Andrews, H. (1991). *The Roy Adaptation Model: The definitive statement*. East Norwalk, CT: Appleton & Lange.

Strauman, J., Frederickson, K., & Jackson, B. (1987). Preliminary report of biopsychosocial effects of Interleukin-2 cancer therapy. *Journal of New York State Nurses Association* 18:50–61.

Part IX

Orem's Self-Care Deficit Theory of Nursing

17

Implementing Self-Care Deficit Nursing Theory: A Process of Staff Development

Katherine McLaughlin

Working with Orem's Self-Care Deficit Nursing Theory (1990, 1991) is very exciting. Before working with this theory, multiple questions came to mind: What is nursing? What is it that nurses do? Why does a person need a nurse? Why should I be a nurse? Self-Care Deficit Nursing Theory (SCDNT) helps answer these questions and clearly differentiates the role of nurse from the role of health educator, social worker, and physician. Clarifying these issues can assist nurses when developing nursing services. For example, opening an office and offering nursing service to the public is made easier by knowing what that service will be. Using Self-Care Deficit Nursing Theory, nursing can be provided without the nurse acting as a mini-doctor and without the patient having an identified medical problem.

Self-Care Deficit Nursing Theory is a theory about nursing practice. The purpose of theory is to help explain nursing and provide direction for practice. The theory helps nurses think 'nursing' and provides for articulation among nursing theories, between nursing knowledge and the knowledge bases of other disciplines, and between nursing theory and related theories.

The process of using Self-Care Deficit Nursing Theory helps nurses think nursing and develop a system of theory-based nursing practice within an organization. The ideas expressed in this chapter stem from my experiences as a student of Self-Care Deficit Nursing Theory, in developing a computerized nursing information system based in the theory, and as a theory resource person for nurses in hospital, community, and educational settings since 1983.

To facilitate staff development in relationship to theory-based practice, each agency I worked with chose to use consultation services rather than project coordinators within the agency for implementing theory-based nursing practice. With no project coordinators to guide implementation, commitment of each nursing manager in the agency was vital to achieving successful implementation.

Theory-based nursing practice means that nurses within a setting use a theory of nursing to provide direction for the design, delivery, and management of nursing programs and services in that organization. All nurses from the Chief Executive Officer of the organization to the new graduate need the theory of nursing integrated into their frame of reference in order to make decisions related to nursing practice. In the following chapter Dale Walker addresses administrative actions which were taken by the Vancouver Health Department to achieve the goals discussed. These administrative actions will now be described as a process of staff development. To clarify, staff development as presented here refers to development of all nurses in an organization, including staff nurses, managers, and the vice-president or president of nursing.

One of the first tasks in an education or staff development program is to determine "what is" in relation to "what is to be accomplished." "What is to be accomplished" is an integration of Self-Care Deficit Nursing Theory into each nurse's frame of reference and using that frame of reference to make nursing decisions. Agreeing with Walker that part of the "what is" is a strong commitment by nurses to the work of nursing; it should be remembered that very few nurses, and others who are responsible for making nursing services available, have a clearly defined conception of what nursing is and why a person needs a nurse. Nursing is generally perceived as a set of tasks to be accomplished. The set of tasks depends on how much money is budgeted for nursing and other services, and how many different health care workers, such as physicians, nurses, physiotherapists, dietitians, and social workers, are available to carry out the tasks.

Integrating Self-Care Deficit Nursing Theory into the decision making frame of reference involves developing an understanding of the proper object of nursing. This involves answering the question: Why does a person need a nurse? The proper object of nursing is the person who is unable to provide over time the quality and quantity of health related self-care which one requires to maintain life, health, integrated functioning, and to promote development. Based on this perspective, nurses need to understand self-care and related concepts of self-care demand, self-care agency, and conditioning factors and their relationships. An additional understanding of designing and delivering nursing systems is necessary for helping or assisting individuals, families, and communities achieve health and well-being.

THE PROCESS AND THE LANGUAGE

The process of helping nurses develop an understanding of these concepts is multifaceted. The concept must have a name, and the first level of resistance is the language associated with the theory.

Is language important? Yes. Why? Let's talk the language of golf: tee off, hole in one, slice, hook, putt, bogey, birdie. Could you talk about golf without using those terms? Let's talk the language of cooking: blend, stir, fold, beat. Are the words as meaningful to non-cooks as to cooks? What language do nurses use? Whose language is appendicitis, blood pressure, colicky pain? These terms represent a body of knowledge which has meaning for nurses, but the meaning is related to the proper object of nursing and nursing theory, the person. For example, the meaning of appendicitis to a physician could be inflammation of the appendix and a need for surgery. Appendicitis to a nurse might mean inflammation of the appendix, a need for surgery, plus a requirement to modify diet and activity following surgery. Hospitalization and illness may also interfere with the process of development, changes in self-care demand, and a requirement for change in self-care agency.

OVERCOMING RESISTANCE TO THE LANGUAGE

Concept Formalization Versus Vocabulary Acquisition

Nurses often object to the language of theory, but the real problem is conceptualizing what the words represent. For example, a lay person who hasn't had a good night's sleep because of awakening every half hour will complain of just that, being awake every half hour for nights on end and being exhausted. In medical language the person may be described as suffering from sleep deprivation. The term sleep deprivation, when used by persons interested in the study of sleep, conjures up a particular picture that is much different from just not getting enough sleep, a very adequate description for the lay person. The term sleep deprivation may be perceived as jargon to the lay person, but it is meaningful language to a medical person. If objection to the language is problematic in concept formalization, the task is to help the person develop an understanding of the concepts represented before language use can begin.

Strategies to Overcome Resistance to Language

First, use the name of the concept. The name eventually should appear in the documentation system if nurses are to collect and analyze data about the concept. The concept name should appear in the performance appraisal tools so that nurses can be evaluated on their abilities to collect and analyze data about the concept. Next, resist the temptation to substitute easier or more common words for the theory concept. For example, when first introduced to Self-Care Deficit Nursing Theory, many persons substitute the term "need" for requisite. Orem has said persons who think this theory has its basis in "need" do not understand the theory. Use the terminology, but take time to explain the concept to nurses. Also, persons responsible for guiding the implementation process must see value in the language as a tool to accomplish a purpose. Use of the language is not an end in itself. The purpose of the language is not to discuss the concerns of nursing with the medical profession, but for nurses to communicate to nurses about the concerns of nursing. Nurses must stop apologizing for having a language which describes the concern of nursing rather than medicine. It is not a case of elitism, it is a necessity.

Just as nurses translate technical language when communicating with patients, some translation is in order when communicating with non-nursing health care workers. When asked whether or not the language of SCDNT interfered with her ability to communicate with physicians, one nurse in the health department stated she believed the language helped her have a clearer picture of what needed to be discussed with the physician and helped clarify the focus and scope of her concern.

CONCEPT ACQUISITION AND STAFF DEVELOPMENT

Concept acquisition as part of a staff development program requires different approaches compared to concept acquisition in nursing education. In nursing education, defining concepts is important, whereas using concepts in practice is as important as being able to recognize when concepts are being used. For example, it is very difficult to define humor. However, humor is often used in nursing practice. In staff development, the goal is to help the staff name what it is they are concerned with and what they are doing. It may be unrealistic to expect staff to define terms in their own words early in the theory implementation process. The ability to define terms represents a very advanced level of understanding and integration that teachers and consultants may have, but not orientees. Staff who are learning to implement Self-Care Deficit Nursing Theory often say, "But we do that." However, they still have difficulty describing for themselves and to others what nursing is and why what they are doing is important. Through implementing appropriate staff development programs, staff can learn to name and identify what it is they are concerned with, what they are doing, and why what they are doing is important.

Part of the process of concept formation and learning about implementing and using Self-Care Deficit Nursing Theory is making the concept explicit in practice. Making the concept explicit in practice is closely tied to the process of learning the language. For example, on a neo-natal intensive care unit in one agency, nurses have established the following committees to examine aspects of their nursing practice: a) consolidation of care, b) positioning and handling, c) environmental control, and d) sensory stimulation. In the language of the Self-Care Deficit Nursing Theory, the nurses are actually focusing on the following requisites of concern: a) balancing rest and activity, b) balancing solitude and social interaction, and c) promotion of development.

Noticing this correlation produces a "teachable moment," an opportunity to make explicit the belief that nurses are acting to meet requisites, coming to know what the requisites are, and forming an action system to accomplish a purpose. It becomes clear for nurses that exchanging the word need for requisite will not work. The manager of the neo-natal unit has chosen this opportunity to help staff nurses see the connections between the committees and requisites by hanging banners in the nursery with the names of the requisites of concern.

On a pediatric unit in our agency, nurses frequently work with adolescent mothers who have great difficulty caring for their children. At a staff meeting, the problem was presented as young mothers who have trouble parenting. Framing the problem from the perspective of Self-Care Deficit Nursing Theory, and using the theory to analyze the situation, the self-care system and the self-care agency of the mothers were found to be inadequate or underdeveloped. After observing the mothers with their children, a relationship was discovered between the degree of development of self-care agency of the mothers and their ability to provide dependent care to their children.

In this instance, using Self-Care Deficit Nursing Theory contributed to several important changes in nursing practice. Theory helped give a new perspective to an old problem. Practitioners became interested in exploring these situations from a research perspective. The concepts of self-care system, self-care agency and dependent-care agency, and dependent care system became real for practicing nurses. Nurses were introduced to an articulation of nursing and family theories focusing on one function of the family, that is, socializing the child into the role of self-care agent (Taylor, 1989). Nurses expanded their role to include helping adolescents develop skills to meet the therapeutic self-care demand for themselves and their children.

During discussions related to this adolescent mother population, socio-cultural orientation was noted as a major conditioning factor in the therapeutic self-care demand of mother and child, and in the development and exercise of self-care and dependent care agency. It became clear that nurses and social workers would need to jointly develop programs and intervention strategies related to this group of patients. Opportunities to discuss and clarify the roles of nurse and social worker emerged from the cooperative effort.

Another strategy for helping staff nurses in the process of concept formalization involves practice based discussions about a particular concept. For example, a staff nurses' study group began by exploring the requisite to maintain a sufficient intake of food. Nurses from various wards shared what this requisite meant for patients on their units and what factors were conditioning the value of and the meeting of the requisite. This discussion helped nurses understand the requisite itself and the relationship of conditioning factors.

In addition to concept acquisition, other benefits from practice-based discussions were observed. As discussions about requisites took place, nurses began to develop standards related to meeting the requisite. The link between use of nursing theory and development of nursing standards was made explicit. It became evident that staff development programs related to nutrition were required, and that tools were needed to help in assessment and documentation. Potential areas for nursing research were identified. The relationship among nursing theory, nursing practice, documentation and nursing research became real. The use of theory was becoming practical for staff nurses.

STAFF DEVELOPMENT AND QUALITY IMPROVEMENT/ASSURANCE PROGRAMS

As theory-based nursing practice is implemented, theory becomes an integral part of the conceptual framework for the definition and evaluation of the quality of nursing practice and nursing services. Organizations usually have a program in place that implements standards for practice and monitors nursing by using a combined medical model and nursing model, with the nursing model being more eclectic than specific. If there is an ongoing program in place which involves staff at many levels throughout the organization, staff development activities should be planned in a variety of ways at all levels.

Several strategies are useful when implementing theory-based nursing practice at many levels in an agency. First, expect vice-presidents and directors of nursing to read the books and articles about the theory written by Dorothea Orem and her colleagues. Expect them to clearly articulate a vision of nursing based in this theory, to share this vision with staff, and to include the nursing staff as an integral part of the nursing decision-making team. Nurses are not born with this vision, it is learned through a process of having opportunities to discuss the theory with peers as a common vision develops. Such discussion ensures congruence between the mission and vision statements of the organization and nursing practice at the bedside.

After deciding to use theory to guide nursing practice, nurses in the organization must explicate how nursing will be practiced in the organization. This activity can be formalized in a written document called "A Guide for Nursing Practice." This guide becomes the reference point for: staff development programs, performance appraisals with reference to nursing practice, development of documentation systems for nursing practice and all other issues related to nursing practice.

Staff and managers must work together to develop a guide that will apply across the agency. Some aspects of the guide will be more pertinent to some clinical areas than others and specific areas can be given the responsibility to develop their own guide. For example, pediatrics and geriatrics are both interested in the dependent care system and evaluation of dependent care agency, although the specific tools related to evaluation may be different.

As nurses participate in developing, testing, and revising the guide, an understanding of the theory and related concepts becomes clarified. The outcome is a standard related to nursing practice which describes expectations in relation to working with the individual (Taylor, 1988), the family (Taylor, 1989), and the community (Taylor & McLaughlin, 1991; McLaughlin & Taylor, in progress). Managers observe their staff and determine variations between practice and the standard. Once objectives are stated, staff development programs can be instituted to help staff meet the standard.

Another strategy is to use elements of the theory to describe characteristics of the populations being served. Descriptions serve as a basis for designing nursing systems for those populations. Developing descriptions is the first step in defining quality indicators for a quality improvement program. This process helps nurses move away from developing quality indicators from a task perspective, such as medication administration. For example, using descriptions assists nurses to think of quality indicators related to helping patients maintain a balance between rest and activity, maintain a balance between solitude and social interaction; and promote normalcy.

When staff work together to develop descriptions, they begin to have a concrete understanding of the relationship between theory and practice. Jointly developed standards relate directly to nursing practice and are more meaningful to nurses at the bedside.

Integrating Self-Care Deficit Nursing Theory into the Decision-Making Framework for Designing In-Service Education Programs

The developed guide for nursing practice is utilized as part of the orientation program. An overview of the practice guide helps new employees understand how nursing is practiced in the agency. Specific questions for discussion include: When is Self-Care Deficit Nursing Theory used for direction? What data are collected and how are those data analyzed? What types of conclusions are drawn? What intervention strategies are available? An introduction to the charting system will also show how theory elements are reflected in the documentation system.

Self-Care Deficit Nursing Theory can organize other classes related to specific nursing technologies. In a class on managing the client on a ventilator, the use of the ventilator is the specific way to meet the requisite of maintaining a sufficient intake of air. However, there are other self-care requisites of concern for the ventilator dependent patient. These minimally include the following: being able to establish and maintain a system of communication, maintaining a balance between rest and activity, maintaining a balance between solitude and social interaction, maintaining a sufficient intake of food and fluid, provision of care related to elimination. In addition, the ability to exercise self-care agency is affected.

Viewed from this perspective, any class related to managing a patient on a ventilator should include information related to the ventilator, a summary of nursing implications, and explorations of changes in the therapeutic self-care demand for these patients. The class content should also explore the affects the ventilator has on the development and exercise of self-care agency and the patient's ability to control his own environment.

Theory gives direction for decision-making about content for staff development and in-service programs. For example, appropriate subject matter could include information to help nurses calculate the therapeutic self-care demand. This includes the process itself and content related to the process. For example, what does sufficient intake of food mean to patients on ventilators? Or what adjustments need to be made in the way the therapeutic self-care demand is met for patients who have had open heart surgery? Note the technique of open heart surgery is not the focus, but the focus is the meaning for the patient variables of therapeutic self-care demand and self-care agency.

As staff work with Self-Care Deficit Nursing Theory, obvious gaps in nursing knowledge appear. A frequent knowledge gap relates to promotion of development in adults. What does this mean? What do we know about developmental processes past the age of twenty? Another common knowledge gap concerns the patient's capabilities associated with the self-care operations of knowing, decision-making, and acting/ doing. What are these capabilities? How do we determine if individuals have developed them and are the capabilities adequate for the current situation?

CONCLUSION

In conclusion, successful implementation of theory-based nursing practice in an organization requires commitment by all nurses in the agency. All nurses must subscribe to a unified way to view the world of nursing. Theory is truly the basis for practice, not something separate and apart.

Theory provides a frame of reference for nursing practice and provides direction for articulation with other theories and knowledge bases. For example, when using Self-Care Deficit Nursing Theory, a nurse may use the work that has been developed by Roy in relation to role, or the body of knowledge related to caring may be accessed.

The view of nursing in an organization guided by the Self-Care Deficit Nursing Theory is demonstrated to all through the integration of theory in the mission/philosophy, the objectives of the nursing department, the orientation program, the staff development programs related to nursing practice, the performance appraisal system, the quality improvement program, and nursing research conducted in the organization.

Staff development processes associated with implementation of theory-based nursing practice are different from those used to teach nursing students how to use theories for direction in their practice. It requires a multifaceted approach which constantly reinforces the use of the selected theory for direction.

Finally, the degree of development of the specific theory selected will influence the implementation processes and may influence the success of the program. When a theory is not well developed, agency staff may not be willing or able to complete the development process.

REFERENCES

McLaughlin, K. E., & Taylor, S. G. (in progress). A directional model for incorporating community focus into nursing process.

Orem, D. E. (1990). A nursing practice theory in three parts, 1956–

1989, in M. Parker (Ed.), *Nursing Theories in Practice*, (pp. 47–60). New York: National League for Nursing Press.

Orem, D. E. (1991). *Nursing: Concepts of practice.* (4th ed.). St. Louis: Mosby.

Taylor, S. G. (1989). An interpretation of family within Orem's general theory of nursing. *Nursing Science Quarterly*, 2, 131–133.

Taylor, S. G. (1988). Nursing theory and nursing process. *Nursing Science Quarterly*, 1, 111–119.

Taylor, S. G., & McLaughlin, K. E. (1991). Orem's general theory and community nursing. *Nursing Science Quarterly*, 4(4), 153–160.

18

A Nursing Administration Perspective on Use of Orem's Self-Care Deficit Nursing Theory

Dale M. Walker

In *Nursing Theories in Practice* (Parker, 1990), the very personal nature of presentations made at previous South Florida Nursing Theorist Conferences is evident. From the preface onward, the authors describe situations that stimulate their personal commitment and willingness to engage in the risk taking behaviors needed to begin the journey into the various worlds of nursing theory and theory-based nursing practice. A nursing administration perspective has value for the implementation of nursing theory. Being a nursing administrator who made a commitment to implement nursing theory into practice, a great personal sense of identification occurred while reading a quote from the chapter written by Vivien Dee (1990) in the first South Florida Theorist Conference book. Dee credits Dorothy Johnson with saying, "To openly use a nursing model is risk-taking behavior for the individual nurse; for a nursing department to adopt one of these models for a unit or institution use is risk-taking behavior of an even higher order" (p. 33). This chapter will outline the major groups of activities undertaken and some risk-taking involved in implementing the Self-Care Deficit Nursing Theory in the Vancouver Health Department, British Columbia, Canada. As well, present and future challenges in theory implementation will be discussed.

Vancouver is a city of 600,000 on the west coast of British Columbia, Canada, 150 miles north of Seattle, Washington. The Vancouver Health Department has 600 staff members with 250 to 300 Community

Health Nurses. Community health nursing services and programs focus on prevention and health promotion, and provide primary care via clinics, home care nursing, and support for seniors and adults with handicapping conditions.

In 1986, the Vancouver Health Department began to explore theory implementation with an eighteen month demonstration project which would identify the system wide impact of implementing Self-Care Deficit Nursing Theory as the basis for nursing practice. The fuel for the project was nurse dissatisfaction and frustration and the will to try new solutions to old problems. Low levels of job satisfaction, continuing greyness of the nursing role, and difficulty in setting priorities for nursing actions and staff education programs were very old problems that we believed could only be overcome by new and probably long term efforts. Upon completion of the project, a decision was made to proceed with full implementation and integration of this nursing theory into practice. We are still in process six years later. Let those faint of heart and conviction not begin on this journey. It has been a major challenge for nurses and administrators to continue with this integration process over six years, amid changing public practices, increasing complexity of community nursing practice, frequently shifting budgets, and other disciplines questioning the value and usefulness of nursing theory for practicing nurses.

This initiative has stimulated many Quality Improvement activities, including revisions of the Philosophy of Community Health Nursing, development of agency Professional Practice Standards, based on the Canadian and British Columbia Nursing Associations' Standards for Nursing Practice (Registered Nurses Association of British Columbia, 1987), and revisions to performance appraisal tools. Activities presenting the most challenge have been revising client record systems and development of ongoing nursing clinical conferences or rounds that support theory based practice—specifically Self-Care Deficit Nursing Theory. These last two activities constituted major undertakings that involved all program supervisors and staff from all nursing units using the theory. Clinical records and nursing conferences describe and support the type, quality, and quantity of nursing generated by the agency; it is imperative that they be useful and useable. Agencies limited to paper record systems are greatly challenged as they face the task of developing staff user-friendly records. If perceived as useful by staff, the record will strongly reinforce the use of nursing theory. If cumbersome and difficult to use, records *become* the nursing theory to the staff. Staff then attribute their frustrations with the record to the theory itself and, thus, fail to benefit from all that Self-Care Deficit Nursing Theory can do to assist them in their practice of nursing. Nursing conferences or rounds have been a most beneficial staff development medium; nurses hear their peers "talk" nursing and learn from each other as they solve problems and gain additional skills in analysis.

CONSIDERATIONS FOR NURSING ADMINISTRATORS

Most senior nurse administrators ask the paramount question, "Should we or should we not adopt a nursing theory in this agency?" Another question might be, "How can we make this agency a more satisfying place to work for more nurses?" Nurses state they cannot practice nursing as they would like because the environments in which they work do not allow professional practice. A dilemma for all!

Mayberry (1991), stresses that the use of theory-based models to guide and direct practice does not require the approval of other professions. She proposes nursing is free to exercise this option on its own authority without a policy decision beyond what nursing decides. Huckaby (1991) notes that the usefulness of nursing theory to the practicing nurse comes from the organization the theory provides for the nurse's thinking, observations, and interpretation of what is seen. Theory provides systematic structure and rationale for activities, points out solutions to practical problems, and provides general criteria for knowing when a problem has been solved. A nurse may strive to practice from a strong and consistent theory base, however, the environment in which she practices will strongly impact her success. Fawcett and Carino (1989) write that nursing practice is mainly controlled by nursing administration. If nursing theory is to rise above sporadic implementation by individual nurses, these authors believe it is essential for nurse administrators to facilitate application of theory on a larger scale.

It seems some authors assert Nursing has the responsibility and the right to make decisions to implement and use nursing theory systemwide, yet other authors believe theory gives structure and substance to individual nursing practice. Nurses are telling nurse administrators to do something, to take action to make the environments in which nurses work more oriented to true caring, skilled nursing. Where do our responsibilities as nursing administrators lie? For those considering implementing nursing theory in their agency, Stevens (1984) poses three questions to consider for the profession in general and nursing administration in particular:

1. Should the administrative structure favor one nursing theory over another?

2. Should different departments or units within the same agency be allowed to select their own theoretical approaches to care delivery?

3. Should nursing administrators perceive theory selection as a right of the individual practitioners and stay out of the theory business?

The opinions and questions raised by Stevens and others who write about issues related to theory implementation are very helpful and worthy of much thought and discussion. The questions offered by Stevens are debated at large and with great feeling in many settings. I have been a part of numerous discussions focusing on one or all of the above commentaries and questions. My position is clear. If nursing theory is to have a consistent impact on nursing care given in any one agency, the selection of one nursing theory is necessary. If nursing theory is to help structure and develop nursing programs and staff education priorities for an agency, the selection of one nursing theory is necessary. On the subject of one theory or many, Dr. Susan Taylor of the University of Missouri-Columbia recommends that administrators ask themselves, "Who do we want to use the theory?" and "What do we want theory to do for the agency?" The questions are helpful in the decision-making process. If the agency wants to use the theory to structure client intake forms on one unit, it may be fine to use more than one nursing theory. It is essential to select one nursing theory if the agency wants theory to guide nurses in the day-to-day complex care of clients, decision-making in nursing practice, supervisors and planners in program development, performance appraisals of staff, and priorities for staff training. This position is based on the belief that nursing administrators have the responsibility to create the structures, systems and forums which facilitate and, indeed, make it possible for nurses to use all their professional and technical skills to benefit clients.

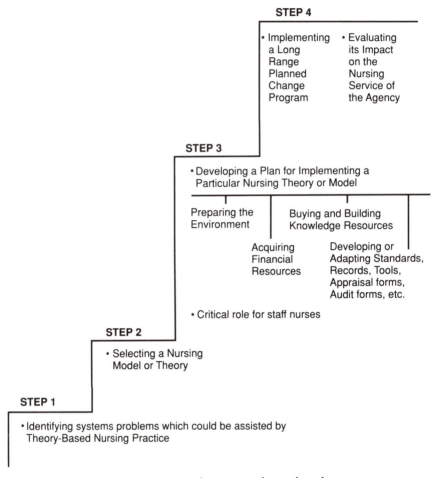

Figure 18.1   Steps in implementing theory-based nursing.

ADMINISTRATIVE ACTIONS

With that as background, the steps taken to implement Self-Care Deficit Nursing Theory in the Vancouver Health Department will be outlined. Figure 18.1 is a representation of the major steps. Although discussion of any one step could be lengthy, this chapter will briefly discuss the individual steps.

Step One: Identifying Systems Problems

Identifying systems problems which could be assisted by theory-based nursing practice is a critical step. All of nursing's problems and issues will not be solved by nursing theory. Even true believers (Oliver, 1991) must admit to that reality! In our department, staff nurses were not satisfied with the degree and type of administrative support given to them while setting priorities and generating directions for clinical decision making. Nursing practice varied from nurse to nurse and unit to unit for the same types of client problems. The literature in 1985 was replete with articles on standards for practice and accountability and staff members were not confident that our agency was practicing accountable nursing. Traditional public health practices were being challenged and nursing roles and practice were under examination. Supervisors were less than confident that their management and supervisory practices were current and were seeking tools to increase their expertise.

Multiple departmental decisions were needed to prepare the system for entrance into the 1990s. Although nursing is part of a multidisciplinary system, senior nurses in the department recognized our primary responsibility was to nursing practice. After numerous discussions, senior nurses came to reasonable consensus: first and foremost, the problems we were experiencing were those we had had for a number of years. Several Band-Aid solutions had been attempted with minimal effect. Secondly, we needed a long range plan that would involve all nursing staff in major ways. Nursing, as the largest discipline in the department, lacked a clear role, a recognizable identity, a strong focus, and direction for the future. The lack of role clarity and professional recognition of nursing within the agency discouraged nurses and contributed to staff unrest. On a positive note, nurses working in patient care oriented areas expressed greater job satisfaction than nurses in education and prevention focus areas. Other strengths included consistent expressions of human and professional caring for the clients by staff, and having nurses who were strongly committed to the work of nursing.

Step Two: Selecting a Nursing Theory

Selecting a nursing theory was not a significant issue at the time we were considering the above problems. Two years previously, a different group of staff made the decision to use Orem's Self-Care Deficit Nursing Theory in the department by using the theory to structure a standards development project. After reviewing several models and theories, the group determined which model would suit the needs of the department. As sometimes happens when people are learning, good ideas cannot be executed because of a lack of know-how. In this case, the project proceeded and the theory stayed comfortably on the proverbial shelf!

Selection of a nursing theory for an agency has been done in three ways. In the first approach, agencies prefer to involve large numbers and all levels of nursing staff in the process. Agencies using this approach often begin with involving staff in values clarification activities, then move to familiarizing themselves with a number of theories in order to select the theory most compatible with their values. This contributes to a smoother implementation process and prepares more nurses prior to the actual implementation of theory into practice. In a second approach, the decision is made by the nursing executive committee or similar group. Nurse executives go through a process of theory selection similar to the first approach, but less time is required due to fewer numbers of people involved. In a third approach, theory selection may be made by the nurse administrator in consultation with staff. The difference in the approaches is the degree of consensus building and, thus, the time required to proceed to implementation. Specific recommendations for taking an agency through the theory selection process can be found in current nursing literature.

Step Three: Planning for Implementation

It is impossible to overemphasize the importance of developing an organized plan for implementation. Introducing Self-Care Deficit Nursing Theory could not have happened in our agency if a strategic plan with a three-year time frame had not been developed. Deadlines had to be extended and postponed. Major in-service programs were postponed time and time again because of service demands, crises of one form or another, or staff resistance. Funds had to be reallocated, staff resigned, but the strategic plan was always there when a renewed sense of direction was needed.

The four major areas for consideration when developing a plan for implementing a nursing theory are: the environment, the financial resource base, the acquisition of knowledge resources, and development of tools for implementation. A detailed account of each area is not possible within the space available in this chapter. Chapters in *Nursing Theories in Practice* (Parker, 1990) outline many of the specifics of nursing theory implementation, and journal articles written since 1986 provide additional information.

Highlights of these major areas are provided so that others may learn from our naivete. First, please expect and plan for resistance! Resistance is important, for it clarifies ideas and the need for theory-based practice. If planned for, resistance is expected, if not expected, its emergence can be terrifying! Rodgers (1989) applied the educational concept of perspective transformation to the evolutionary learning process which nurses undergo as they learn nursing theory. In the chapter on educating nurses in the Self-Care Deficit Nursing Theory, (Chapter 17), Katherine McLaughlin has discussed that process in some detail.

Secondly, acquiring and allocating financial resources requires decisions, difficult decisions that can only be made by nursing administrators. Controlling significant budgets and having the ability to allocate funds are definite advantages. If nurse administrators do not have these abilities, they must look for creative and innovative ways to make the administrative changes which will permit professional practice. Nurse administrators make decisions, everyday decisions, which reflect their understanding of and support for the professional practice of nursing. Financial support is needed for theory implementation, and resource allocation is the prerogative of most nurse administrators. Nurse administrators insure nursing care given in an agency is, in fact, nursing, and that the quality of nursing care is satisfactory to the community. In all agencies, nursing requires resources that are acquired and allocated by nursing administrators. How do nurse administrators make decisions about resources? Many agencies choose a model or theory, then discover resources are not available to support the decision to implement the theory into practice. Perhaps nurse administrators need to re-think and define how and why allocation decisions are made. Are they using decision-making habits that are hard to break?

A third area involves buying and building knowledge resources and educational supports for implementing nursing theory. Preparing for theory implementation is greatly enhanced if educational resources are available and can be purchased rather than produced. Availability of self-learning and educational materials for group teaching is of paramount importance. Agency-wide theory based practice is a future-oriented undertaking that requires considerable advanced planning and a long range vision and plan to be successful, yet practical, in its execution. Acquiring staff with advanced skills in nursing practice is a constant challenge for nurse managers and administrators. Acquiring staff with these skills and with sufficient leadership experience to both plan and execute a program of system-wide theory implementation is very difficult. Although there is much supporting rhetoric that hails the benefits of nursing theory for practice, there are few nurses with experience in agency-wide theory implementation. It is, therefore, most practical and time efficient to begin planning at the outset how the agency will develop these skills in the staff already employed in the agency. To a large extent, the education levels of the agency senior nursing staff will dictate the resources which can be developed in-house and those which the agency will want to purchase. Currently, an increasing number of teaching materials can be purchased and it is possible to hire knowledgeable consultants to assist in the implementation process.

The last of four areas to be discussed under the steps of developing the plan is developing the tools for implementation. Tool development is viewed as a significant undertaking and in our experience, it was! Few resources for implementing Self-Care Deficit Theory of Nursing were available at the time we began, and those that were available were difficult to adapt to the needs of a community health agency. We developed the philosophy, assessment tools, standards, orientation manuals and appraisal tools, in a manner similar to those being reported in current literature. In addition, all tools have undergone several changes during the six years since we began.

These changes have been a source of some concern and displeasure to those who, through experience, had come to expect that forms, once developed, would stay unchanged for many, many years. In today's world, that expectation is a "sacred cow." That "sacred cow," along with many others, is being replaced quickly. "New calves" take their place and they will not likely see adolescence. Nursing will continue to change rapidly in the next decade. The resources and tools which help shape nursing practice in agencies will have to change along with nursing practice if they are to help and not hinder our efforts to bring more professional practice to populations requiring nursing.

Step Four: Implementing and Evaluating
the Program of Theory Implementation

A process of planning for a long range change process has been discussed. Identifying theory implementation as a separate, major step may seem redundant, however, it is done to underscore implementation as another critical stage in the process. It is a long range undertaking that, if successful, has the power to forever change how nursing will be practiced in individual agencies. This is the hope we hold for our agency. As every year passes, and more staff develop expertise in using the concepts of Self-Care Deficit Nursing Theory of Nursing to assist them in analyzing the complex client situations they face every day, I become more convinced that implementation of theory will bring long lasting changes to nursing practice in the agency.

At the outset of the chapter, it was noted that six years have elapsed since the introduction of Self-Care Deficit Nursing Theory began in our agency. There have been many delays along the way. Experiences of other agencies have been similar. The challenge is to keep the process going! Initial evaluation data obtained in 1986–1987 and 1988–1990 maintain the forward movement of the process. The data indicate that nurses learning to use this theory are able to see as many clients during a month as those not learning the theory. Work load is not negatively affected. The majority of staff can use the new record system with reasonable facility within six months following the introduction of the theory to a unit. There is a demonstrated need for additional support to increase skill in using the new system, and we are prepared to provide that support. Some staff say the new system makes no difference in their ability to identify client problems, but others believe the system helps them more clearly identify when to admit and discharge clients. It becomes easier for staff to determine when there is a requirement for nursing, or when clients require assistance of another discipline. According to Orem's Self-Care Deficit Nursing Theory (1991), a person is in need of or can benefit from nursing when there is a deficit in his ability to provide the quantity or quality of self-care needed for satisfactory functioning. Evaluation data gave direction for making changes and gave the initial credibility needed to sustain the continuation of funding.

Evaluation, that is informal evaluation, is ongoing. As an agency where service delivery is the mandate, funding and personnel resources for formal evaluation are limited. Also, few nurses have expertise in research, therefore, changes in practice are usually based on informal evaluation and staff feedback. Selected supervisors and managers are beginning to see how concepts and relationships of Self-Care Deficit Nursing Theory can structure studies looking at client populations' needs for nursing based on common types and numbers of self-care deficits. Using theory can lead to more informed considerations for targeting specific populations with particular self-care deficits and environmental risks, and when proposing population specific interventions. For example, environmental risks which make adequate self-care impossible could include unsafe and inadequate living conditions, eating from food lines, using unsafe injection practices, or unsafe sex practices.

Our staff would like to develop research expertise and ongoing resources so that clinical research can be conducted with specific client populations. A group is preparing to address this challenge in 1992, as we move to establish a research committee that will bring in outside research expertise from the professional association and interested university schools of nursing. The challenge is to interest non-agency research experts to conduct research in the areas of interest to us, an agency moving on with the implementation of Self-Care Deficit Theory of Nursing.

In summary, the challenges have been many and will continue. There are significant differences now in who responds to the challenges. At one time it was my role to defend the values of nursing theory in the agency. Now the supervisors and many of the nursing staff come forward to support why it is important to continue the work we have begun. It is very exciting to watch this happen. It has been and continues to be an exciting challenge to assist nurses to develop so they can speak with confidence, identify nursing requirements of clients, and clearly articulate the role of nursing and the role of nursing theory in their practice.

REFERENCES

Dee, V. (1990). Implementation of the Johnson model: One hospital's experience. In M. Parker (Ed.), Nursing Theories in Practice. New York: National League for Nursing Press.

Fawcett, J. (1989). Analysis and evaluation of conceptual models of nursing. (2nd ed.). Philadelphia, PA: Davis.

Fawcett, J., & Carino, C. (1989). Hallmarks of success in nursing practice. Advances in Nursing Science. 11(4), 1–8.

Huckaby, L. (1991). The role of conceptual frameworks in nursing practice, administration, education and research. Nursing Administration Quarterly, 15(3), 17–28.

Mayberry, A. (1991). Merging nursing theories, models and nursing practice: More than an administrative challenge. *Nursing Administration Quarterly*, 15(3), 44–53.

Oliver, N. R. (1991). True believers: A case for model-based nursing practice. *Nursing Administration Quarterly*, 15(3), 37–43.

Orem, D. (1991). *Nursing: Concepts of practice*. (4th ed.). St. Louis: Mosby.

Parker, M. (Ed.) (1990). *Nursing Theories in Practice*. New York: National League for Nursing Press.

Registered Nurses Association of British Columbia. (1987). *Standards for Nursing Practice in British Columbia*. Vancouver: Registered Nurses Association of British Columbia.

Rodgers, B. (1989). Concept analysis and the development of nursing knowledge: The evolutionary cycle, *Journal of Advanced Nursing*. 14(4), 330–335.

Stevens, B. J. (1984). *Nursing theory: Analysis, application, evaluation*. (2nd ed.) Boston: Little, Brown.

Part X

The Johnson Behavioral System Model

19

The Johnson Behavioral System Model: Perspectives for Nursing Practice

Anayis K. Derdiarian

This chapter, and the one following, explore application of the Johnson Behavioral System (JBS) Model (Johnson, 1980, 1990) in nursing practice. The application of any nursing model to practice requires three conditions: the model's congruence with practice requirements, its comprehensive development in relation to practice requirements, and its specificity in relation to practice requirements. These conditions governing a nursing model's applicability should be understood to enable practitioners to appropriately and effectively use models in practice.

The purpose of this chapter is to present three segments: practice requirements, conditions for the Model's applicability including instrumentation, and the applicability of the JBS Model to nursing practice. What is nursing practice and what are requirements of this practice? Nursing practice derives its definition from that of professional practice, the action or process of performing something, the habitual or customary performance of something (Random House College Dictionary, 1988). Professional practice has three main requirements: perspective, structure, and scientific substance.

PERSPECTIVE FOR NURSING PRACTICE

The first requirement is the perspective, or a mental view, of facts or ideas and their interrelationships pertinent to the profession's practice.

In nursing, the perspective of the practice refers to nursing's view of the patient and its role in relation to the patient. More specifically, the profession's perspective clarifies the *nature, goal, focus,* and *scope* of its realm of its science and practice (Derdiarian, 1991). By so doing, the profession's perspective distinguishes nursing's realm of science and practice from those of related fields. At the same time, the perspective identifies appropriate alignments between nursing's research and practice and those of other professions. In other words, the professional perspective provides the professional with a knowledge base and a mind-set about the patient, about her/his role in relation to the patient, and her/his actions necessary to fulfill that role.

Consistent with the professional perspective, the *nature* of practice refers to the qualities or characteristics of the scientific content that underlies practice. In nursing, this content is the facts, knowledges, phenomena, and assumptions about the patient that nursing shares with other related professions, but in a uniquely different way, and for a uniquely different purpose. Nature of practice answers the question, what facts, knowledges, phenomena, assumptions, and beliefs does nursing use, and in what priority or relationship does it use them to rationalize its practice? The *goal* of a profession's practice is the end-result it attempts to achieve in the patient. In nursing, the goal is the state or condition in the patient that nursing intends to achieve as a result of its practice. In other words, what are the patient outcomes nursing purports to claim as its own product?

The *focus* of a profession's practice refers to the areas or points of practice to which the professional directs particular attention. In nursing, the foci of practice are the ills it aims to fix or alleviate. In practical terms, these ills are the types of problems nursing intends to solve. Finally, the *scope* of a profession is its conceptual borders, encompassing its perspective of the patient, its role in relation to that perspective, the range of its foci, and the range of its actions and processes. In nursing, the *scope* pertains to boundaries of its view of the patient, its role in relation to the patient, the range of the problems focal to its practice, and the range of actions it takes to solve the problems. In more practical terms, the scope of practice pertains to the comprehensiveness of the view of the patient's well-being as well as of the problems and their solutions.

Structure for Practice

The second requirement of professional practice is a structure for practice to organize and standardize practice and, thus, render practice habitual and customary. Professional practice is structured to evaluate a patient's well-being, identify problems, and provide solutions. The latter require organized and scientifically rational processes of assessment, diagnosis, intervention, and evaluation of outcomes. In nursing, this structure pertains to the Nursing Process.

Scientific Substance for Practice

Finally, the third requirement of professional practice is the coherent scientific body of knowledge that underlies it or the profession's actions and processes. The scientific body of knowledge includes facts, theories, hypotheses, and precepts, and assumptions underlying both the perspective and structure of practice. In nursing, this body of knowledge includes the facts, theories, hypotheses, and precepts about nursing, nursing practice actions, and nursing practice methods. Stated more specifically, nursing practice requires verifiable knowledge that rationalizes its view of the patient, its role, nature, goal focus, and scope. Furthermore, nursing practice requires a body of scientific knowledge that rationalizes the nursing methods of assessment, diagnosis, intervention, and evaluation of outcomes. The foregoing section summarizes the essential requirements of professional practice. A related and equally important requirement is the model's social acceptability within the scientific, professional, economic, and consumeristic parameters of practice (Derdiarian, 1990).

CONDITIONS FOR NURSING MODELS' APPLICABILITY TO PRACTICE

The applicability of a nursing model, in this case the JBS model, depends upon three conditions: its congruence with practice requirements, the degree of its development in relation to practice requirements, and lastly, the degree of its specification to practice requirements. These conditions are reviewed and amplified as follows.

Congruence with Practice

Congruence with practice requirements means the model corresponds identically with the practice requirements. Said differently, when superimposed, the model should coincide with all the requirements of practice, which are the professional perspective for practice, the structure for practice, and the scientific substance that underlies the perspective and structure of professional practice. Thus, in relation to the JBS model, this condition raises the question, Is the JBS model congruent with the practice requirements?

Development Sufficient for Specification for Practice

Comprehensive Development refers to the degree to which the model's conceptual development is sufficiently complete, to render it congruent with all the points of practice requirements. More specifically, Does the model clearly identify a perspective for nursing practice, a structure for nursing practice, and a scientific body of knowledge that underlies the perspective and structure for practice? If not sufficiently developed, does the model point to the areas and degrees of development required to render its development sufficiently complete in relation to the practice requirements? Said more simply, Do the theorist and/or the followers point to or develop the areas of the model requiring further development for proper application to practice? This condition compels the question, Is JBS model sufficiently developed to ensure its congruence with practice requirements?

Specification Sufficient for Applicability to Practice

Specification to practice requirements refers to a model's reduction to the various levels of specificity needed to render it operational or applicable in practice. An example of the levels of specification of one of the model's concepts, Achievement, is demonstrated in Figure 19.1.

Most, if not all, nursing models in their current stage of development, are in their conceptual stage. As such, they represent a coherent set of facts, ideas, precepts, hypotheses, assumptions, and beliefs that represent their respective authors' proposed views about or for nursing. Although an essential step, in their current state of development, these nursing models grossly lack the necessary steps of specification to become operational in practice. These specifications should include adequate conceptual development, theoretical specification, methodological specification, empirical specification, and clinical specification, as demonstrated in the Columns 1 through 6 respectively, in Figure 19.1. In relation to the JBS model, this condition poses the question, Is the JBS model specified to nursing practice requirements? Collectively, the

SUBSYSTEM CONCEPT →	THEORETICAL SPECIFICATION →	METHODOLOGICAL SPECIFICATION →	EMPIRICAL SPECIFICATION →	CLINICAL SPECIFICATION →	APPLICATION IN NURSING PROCESS →
Achievement	1. Ability to achieve	1. Ability to pursue goals - Ability to perform - (Six other items)	Psychometric and Clinical data base supporting the DBSM and DBSM-O Instrument items	Data Base Supporting DBSM and DBSM-O to guide assessment data generation required to diagnose and intervene in nursing problems	- Assessment data - Analysis of data - Interpretation of data, identification of type of behavior
	2. Incentive to achieve	2. Importance of planning goals - Importance of pursuing goals - Importance of performance - (Five other items)			- Nursing Diagnosis - Nursing Goal/Patient Outcome - Identification of appropriate type of nursing interventions
	3. Spiritual strength or hope to achieve	3. Spiritual strength to achieve goals - Hope to achieve goals - (Five other items)			- Evaluation

Figure 19.1 An excerpt demonstrating the steps of process of specifying the Johnson Behavioral System Nursing Model from concept to application to nursing process, using the Achievement Subsystem.

foregoing questions ask, Is the JBS model applicable to nursing practice? To answer these questions, the JBS model is reviewed and evaluated against the conditions of a model's applicability to practice.

APPLICABILITY OF JBS MODEL TO NURSING PRACTICE REQUIREMENTS

The earlier identified practice requirements are perspective for practice, structure for practice, and scientific body of knowledge to underlie practice and its methods. The JBS model, in its original form, meets this set of practice requirements to a large extent, as discussed below.

Perspective for Practice. The JBS model proposes a perspective for nursing practice by viewing the human as a bio-psycho-social being represented in a behavioral system that is comprised of seven behavioral subsystems (SSs) or behavioral components. The behavioral SSs are Achievement, Aggressive/Protective, Affiliative, Dependency, Ingestive, Eliminative, and Sexual. An eighth SS, the Restorative SS, was proposed by followers of Johnson. Most applications of the model including mine have included the eighth SS. Humans meet the demands of life based on the effective functioning of the behavioral SSs which result in a behavioral system balance. The SSs are viewed as being interactive and interdependent. Illness is viewed as introducing disruption to the system's behavioral balance. The disruption may be manifested in one or more SSs and it affects the behavioral system balance. Nursing's *role* is to help the patient maintain or regain behavioral system integrity required for the restoration of health and function. The *nature* of nursing is identified as the integrity of the behavioral functioning of the SSs, especially after illness. The *goal* for nursing is the restoration and maintenance of behavioral balance in the system to the greatest extent possible. The *focus* for nursing practice is the identification and restoration of ineffective behavioral response to illness. The *scope* of nursing practice entails the conceptual boundaries outlined by the seven behavioral SSs or components. Each behavioral SS has its own substructure: set, drive, goal, choice, and action. *Set* refers to the individual's propensity to behave in relation to the SS goal in a given situation. It is affected by genetic, developmental, and environmental factors. *Drive* is based in human need and it energizes behavior toward the achievement of goal or fulfillment of need. *Choice* refers to the behavior selected and *action* refers to behavior observed. It is the paper's contention, that the range of behavioral disruptions, and therefore the ineffective behavioral responses to illness, would occur within the *scope* of the model. Accordingly, the range of nursing diagnostic and interventive activities could be contained within the model's SSs. The range of behavioral disruptions could include intra-SS problems, or SS structural problems and inter-SS problems or SS inter-actional problems. The range of such problems could vary because the behavioral SSs are interactive and interdependent; therefore, disruption in one could help predict disruption in another or others. Conversely, because the SSs are interactive and interdependent, restoration of behavior in one SS could effect restoration of behavior in another or others. Therefore, the *scope* for practice implies that the comprehensive care of the patient requires diagnostic and interventive actions directed at all of the SSs. Thus, the JBS model meets the professional perspective requirements well.

Structure for Practice. The JBS model proposes a conceptual structure for nursing practice. Consistent with the model's perspective of the goal and foci of practice, the generic nature of patients' problems, or the behavioral imbalance is specified to a typology of patient problems. The model identifies the typology of patient problems as Insufficiency, Dominance, Incompatibility, and Discrepancy. The implication here is that patient's behavioral problems, or nursing diagnoses of these problems could belong to one of these types. Therefore, ineffective behavior should be analyzed as to its problematic type or identity. *Insufficiency* type refers to the inadequacy of the behavior to achieve the goal of the SS in order to regain health or function due to insufficient functional requirement for the behavior's development and sustenance. *Dominance* type refers to the excessive behavior not warranted or counteractive to achieve the goal. Discrepancy type refers to the inconsistency of the chosen action or behavior with set, or drive, or goal. And, *Incompatibility* type refers to the behavior aimed at achieving a SS goal that is incompatible with another behavior aimed at achieving another SS goal.

It can be extrapolated from the model that, as a result of illness any of the above types of problems could occur in one or more of the behavioral SSs. Thus, the JBS model points to areas for assessment, identifies problems to assess, and provides a typology to categorize the problems.

Similarly, the JBS model provides a conceptual structure to guide and organize nursing interventive actions. Again consistent with the model's goal for nursing action, the model identifies a typology of nursing interventions. Because the generic nature of nursing intervention is SS behavioral integrity and behavioral system balance, the model identifies five types of interventions—Nurturance, Stimulation, Protection, Regulation, and Control. *Nurturance* type interventions aim at promoting development of appropriate behavior needed to achieve a desired goal by providing nourishment, support, and encouragement. *Stimulation* type interventions intend to arouse or activate dormant or passive patient behaviors to achieve desired goals. *Protection* type interventions pursue defending or guarding appropriate patient behavior from attack, loss, insult, injury, or harm. *Regulation* type interventions aim at directing or controlling patient behavior by a rule, principle, or method prescribed by authority. Finally, *Control* type interventions intend to restrain or dominate ineffective patient behavior based on professional judgment, purpose, and standard.

A close examination of the typology of problems and interventions reveals an interesting and important relationship among them. There seems to be a specificity of relationships between the types of problems and types of interventions. For example, it is plausible that insufficiency type problems may be more appropriately influenced by Nurturance type interventions. Dominance type problems could more effectively be dealt with by Control type interventions. Incompatibility type and discrepancy type problems could be better solved by stimulation, regulation, and control types of interventions respectively.

This discussion of the JBS model demonstrates its congruence with the practice structure requirements. Although not in appreciable specificity, the model does suggest where to look for problems, what to assess and diagnose, and how to intervene in those problems. It should be noted, that the model does not identify methods or means for practice. That is, the model does not identify how to assess and intervene.

Scientific Substance for Practice.   The third and final set of practice requirements relates to the scientific substance that underlies the model's perspective, practice, and methods. The model's perspective and practice structure are founded in the biological, medical, and behavioral sciences. Although not readily verifiable, the models' major concepts and propositions are potentially verifiable through scientific testing. For example, the SSs, their substructures and their interaction and interdependence are theoretically sound. That the integrity of behavioral SS function is essential for total system function to sustain health and function is also theoretically sound. Also, that illness introduces disruption to behavioral balance through disruption in one or more SSs is theoretically sound. That behavioral imbalance expressed as potentially or actually ineffective behavioral response in one SS or another and, if not addressed could cause behavioral disruptions or ineffective responses in others is theoretically sound. That the SSs could provide adequate boundaries to contain the ranges of behavioral disruptions could be theoretically verifiable. Finally, the specificity of relationships between the behavioral disruptions and their effective treatments could be verified. That the behavioral disruptions could be categorized in the four types is theoretically plausible. Also, that intervention types could be categorized in the four types is theoretically defensible.

One of the most scientifically unique features of this model is the model's definitions of the *drive* and *goal* of each SS. These definitions help to conceptualize and define the SS concepts in mutually exclusive ways. This feature is of utmost importance for concept analysis, measurement, and application to practice. The natural question is, Are the above conjectures true? The answer is, they need to be tested.

As noted above, the JBS does not provide scientific substance in relation to the methods of assessment, diagnosis, intervention and evaluation of outcomes of practice. However, because the model's conceptual framework identifies nursing problems and actions, methods for diagnostic and interventive actions could be extrapolated from it.

Recapping the evaluation of the JBS model in relation to Practice Requirements, it is evident that this model meets the Practice Perspective and Practice Structure Requirements well. It does not meet well the Scientific Substance Requirements primarily because it needs scientific testing of its concepts, propositions, and assumptions outlined above. Furthermore, it needs to provide scientific methods for its practice procedures. The scientific testing of the model and the scientific development of its method are connected with the third condition of applicability, the model's specification to practice.

Conditions for Applicability

Evaluating the JBS model in relation to the conditions of practice, the following conclusion can be reached.

Congruence and Development Sufficient for Practice Requirements. In the previous discussion, it is clear that the JBS model has an overall congruence with the Practice Requirements and, therefore, it generally meets the applicability to practice requirement. The model lacks points to match the important points of methods of practice, namely, the methods of assessment, diagnosis, intervention, and evaluation of outcomes.

Also in the previous discussion, it is evident that the JBS model is generally well developed in relation to the Practice Requirements. As in relation to the condition of congruence, the model requires development to provide the methods of practice—theoretical, methodological, empirical, and clinical.

Specification to Practice Requirements. In its original state, the JBS is not specified to provide the scientific substance to its perspective, structure for practice, and methods of practice. The ensuing presentation demonstrates the stages and procedures undertaken (Derdiarian, 1983; Derdiarian and Forsythe, 1983) to render the JBS model applicable to practice.

Theoretical Specification: The ultimate questions to be answered were the following.

> Is there scientific evidence to support the model's perspective about the patient? If there is, what are the theoretical elements that substantiate the conceptual structure and processes of this model's perspective?

Expressed in more scientific statements, the above question contains the following research questions:

1. What are the scientific elements, concepts, or factors of the SSs behavioral system?

2. Are these elements measurable or verifiable?

3. Do changes occur in the SSs as a result of illness?

4. Do the SSs provide comprehensive boundaries to detect behavioral changes resulting from illness?

5. Are the SSs interactive?

Therefore, the initial work focused on concept analysis and theoretical construct development to specify each of the major concepts constituting the model—the SSs, behavioral balance change, comprehensiveness of the system's boundaries, and inter subsystem interaction. The work included exploring the appropriate scientific literature and developing the concepts theoretically, or finding theoretical substantiation for the concepts. What are the theoretical elements of the SSs? Does the theoretical literature support the model's propositions of behavioral system change, system boundaries, and SS interaction? The literature review was guided by the model's definitions of its concepts and propositions. Each SS's definition of its *drive* and *goal* provided direction to identify, understand, and substantiate the theoretical elements of each SS as an individual theoretical entity. It was evident that each behavioral SS had its biophysical and psychosocial determinants in the scientific literature. The theoretical construction of the model yielded a theoretical structure of the model outlined in the first column of Table 19.1.

The literature indicated some theoretical support for the model's propositions 2, 3, 4 (Derdiarian, 1983; Derdiarian and Forsythe, 1983), and 5 (Derdiarian, 1991). This theoretical form of the model moved it from its conceptual or phenomenological state to its more specific and theoretical state. The question is, Is the model now more scientific and applicable in its theoretical state? The answer is, it is more scientific and more applicable, but not sufficiently so. A broader and more specified perspective does not prove scientific and applicational value. This realization moved the work toward the second state—the methodological specification of the model.

Methodological Specification: The theoretically specified structure of the model needed to be further specified to become measurable or verifiable based on scientific methods. Therefore, each concept should be made measurable. Thus, each concept construct was defined in operational or measurable terms (or empirical referents, or measurable items), (Derdiarian, 1983).

The question is, Is this form or state of the model more scientifically relevant and applicable? The answer is, the model is relatively more scientific and applicable than its former status, but its scientific value has not yet been tested or demonstrated. Therefore, the model should move to its empirical state. This means scientific data are required to demonstrate its scientific relevance and applicability. The processes applied to further reduce the model are outlined in the following section.

Table 19.1   Behavioral System Model for Nursing Practice as Theoretically Developed and Specified in Subsystems and Categories

SUBSYSTEM AND CATEGORY AS DEFINED BY DBSM	GOALS AS DEFINED BY THE JOHNSON MODEL
Achievement 1. Ability (physical and mental) to achieve 2. Incentive to achieve 3. Hope or belief in God's help to achieve	To master self or environment; to achieve mastery and control.
Affiliation 1. Relating to one's own beliefs, God, or Spiritual Being 2. Relating to one's family, close friends, or relatives 3. Relating to one's job or social acquaintances	To relate or belong to something or someone other than oneself; to achieve intimacy and inclusion.
Aggressive/protective 1. Possessing physical stamina (or reserve) 2. Possessing cognitive stamina 3. Possessing emotional stamina	To protect self or others from real or imagined threatening objects, persons, or ideas; to achieve self-protection and self-assertion.
Dependence 1. Physical reliance on others or objects 2. Cognitive reliance on others or objects 3. Emotional reliance on others or objects	To maintain environmental resources needed for obtaining help, attention, permission, reassurance and security; to gain trust and reliance.
Eliminative 1. Gastrointestinal elimination 2. Genitourinary elimination 3. Integumentary, lacrimal, and other elimination	To expel biologic wastes; to externalize the internal biologic environment.

Table 19.1   Continued

SUBSYSTEM AND CATEGORY AS DEFINED BY DBSM	GOALS AS DEFINED BY THE JOHNSON MODEL
Ingestive	
1. Food and fluid intake 2. Food and fluid retention/ assimilation 3. Psychosocial determinants of eating	To take in needed resources from the environment to maintain integrity of the organism or to achieve a state of pleasure.
Restorative	
1. Sleep 2. Relaxation/recreation 3. Physiologic	To relieve fatigue and/or achieve a state of equilibrium by reestablishing the energy distribution among the other subsystems; to redistribute energy.
Sexual	
1. Gender identity 2. Physical sexual functioning 3. Psychosocial sexual functioning	To procreate, to gratify or attract, to fulfill expectations associated with gender; to care for others and be cared about by others.

Empirical Specification: This stage involved gathering scientific data to substantiate the validity of the SSs' theoretical constructs; it also involved the propositions that behavioral balance changes occur as a result of illness, that the SSs provide adequate boundaries to contain the changes, and that the SSs are interactive.

Behavioral balance change was measured as a patient's perceived changes in the SS behavior construct elements or categories. And change was measured by the amount or degree of change (increase or decrease), quality (positive or negative or relative impact, importance value 1 to 100), and causal or associational factors (effects of illness), (Derdiarian and Forsythe, 1983).

The data gathered from several large samples of adult cancer patients support the validity of the theoretical constructs of the SSs as well as the propositions of behavioral change, system boundaries (Derdiarian, 1991), and SS interaction (Derdiarian, 1991). Repeated content validation by experts, as well as construct validation methods using patient profile analysis and factor analysis methods have very strongly supported the model's empirical specification (Derdiarian, 1988). The reliability of this specification was also supported by repeated test-retest and internal consistency methods (Derdiarian and Forsythe, 1983). Data also supported direct and indirect relationships between and among the SSs (Derdiarian, 1990). See Figures 19.2 and 19.3.

The compelling question is, Is the model as empirically tested more scientifically relevant and applicable to practice? The answer is yes, more so now than in its former forms. The model now has scientific reference but, Is it clinically applicable? Does the model now meet the practice requirements to guide and underlie the nursing process? The answer is, not just yet. Therefore, the final stage of specification of

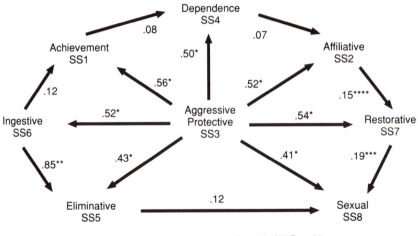

*P <.001, **P <.002, ***P <.02, ****P <.05

Reprinted from *Image: Journal of Nursing Scholarship*, with permission of Sigma Theta Tau International, Inc., Derdiarian, Anayis K., The Relationships Among the Subsystems of Johnson's Behavioral System Model. *Image*, vol. 22, (4), 1990, pp. 219–225.

Figure 19.2 Significant relationships among the subsystems from increase/decrease scale outcomes.

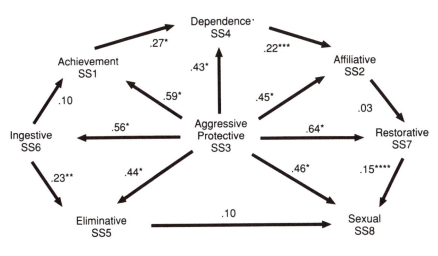

*P <.001, **P <.003, ***P <.005, ****P <.06

Reprinted from *Image: Journal of Nursing Scholarship*, with permission of Sigma Theta Tau International, Inc., Derdiarian, Anayis K., The Relationships Among the Subsystems of Johnson's Behavioral Systems Model. *Image*, vol. 22, (4), 1990, pp. 219–225.

Figure 19.3 Significant relationships among the subsystems from positive/negative scale path analysis outcomes.

the model was to make it suitable for the nursing process application. The following section outlines the procedures and outcomes of this final stage of the model's specification.

Clinical Specification: Once data support validation and patient relevancy of the DBSM instrument were established, an objective instrument was needed to meet the nursing process requirements. Therefore, a Behavioral Observational instrument was needed to gather observational data alongside the subjective or self-reported data from the DBSM instrument. This development would have the added value of testing the DBSM instrument's clinical applicability. Therefore, the DBSM observational instrument (DBSM-O) was developed. From the operational definitions of the model's theoretical constructs, the DBSM-O items were constructed based on the scientific biomedical and behavioral sciences. For each item of the DBSM, five to six behavioral/observational, medical, instrumentational, and laboratory measures were identified as appropriate. The DBSM-O's content-validity and in-

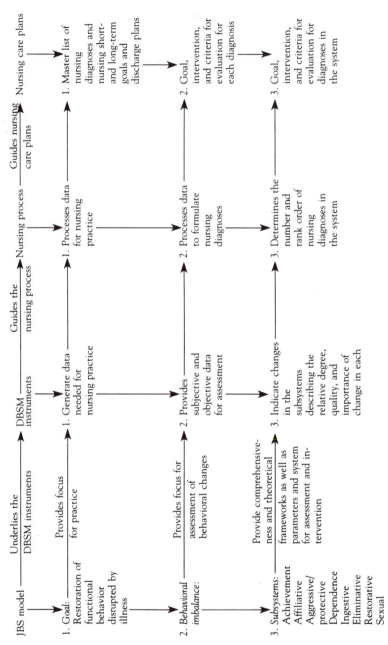

Figure 19.4 The relationship of the JBS (Johnson Behavioral System) Model to the nursing process.

Reprinted from the *Oncology Nursing Forum* with permission from the Oncology Nursing Press, Inc., Derdiarian, Anayis K., The Effects of Using Systematic Assessment Instruments on Patient and Nurse Satisfaction with Nursing Care, *Oncology Nursing Forum* 17(1):95–101, 1990. Also reprinted in *Nursing Administration Quarterly*, Vol. 15, No. 3, p. 6, with permission of Aspen Publishers, Inc., copyright 1991.

ter-rater reliability were tested. It served as the source of objective data needed to do assessments and reassessments of a patient's problems as a counterpart to the DBSM, the source for the subjective data. Based on the DBSM and DBSM-O data, a patient's problem(s) in each of the SS were identified, diagnosed, and classified. Nursing care plans addressing each problem were developed and implemented, and outcomes were evaluated. The study's results on the comprehensiveness and quality of the nursing process implementation (Derdiarian, 1991), nurse-satisfaction and patient-satisfaction with the nursing practice were demonstrated as being directly related to the model's application to the nursing process (Derdiarian, 1988, 1989). Therefore, it was demonstrated that the JBS Model achieved clinical specification and, thus, clinical applicability. The final questions are: Did the JBS Model achieve scientific support to underlie its perspective for nursing and to underlay its method for the nursing process? The answer is that it did. The process of specifying the model from its conceptual to its clinical applicability is outlined in Figure 19.4.

The foregoing analysis and evaluation of the JBS Model's inception, development, and testing in relation to the conditions of a model's applicability demonstrate that this model is applicable to practice.

REFERENCES

Derdiarian, A. K. (1983). An instrument for research and theory development using the Behavioral System Model for Nursing: The cancer patient. Part I. *Nursing Research*, 32:4, 196–201.

Derdiarian, A. K. (1988). Sensitivity of the Johnson Behavioral System Model for nursing practice instrument to age, site and stage of cancer: A preliminary validation study. *Scholarly Inquiry for Nursing Practice*, 2:2, 103–120.

Derdiarian, A. K. (1990). The effects of using systematic assessment instruments on patient and nurse satisfaction. *Oncology Nursing Forum*, 17:1, 95–101.

Derdiarian, A. K. (1991). Effects of using a nursing model-based assessment instrument on quality of nursing care. *Nursing Administration Quarterly*, 15:3, 1–16.

Derdiarian, A. K. (1991). The relationships among the subsystems of

Johnson's Behavioral System Model. *Image: Journal of Nursing Scholarship*, 22:4, 219–225.

Derdiarian, A. K., & Forsythe, A. W. (1983). An instrument for research and theory development using the Behavioral System Model for Nursing: The cancer patient. Part II. *Nursing Research*, 32:5, 260–265.

Johnson, D. E. (1980). The behavioral system model of nursing. In J. Riehl and C. Roy (Eds.). *Conceptual Models for Nursing Practice* (2nd ed.), (pp. 207–216). New York: Appleton-Century-Crofts.

Johnson, D. E. (1990). The behavioral system model for nursing. In M. Parker (Ed.). *Nursing Theories in Practice* (pp.23–32). New York: National League for Nursing Press.

Random House College Dictionary, 1988.

20

Application of the Johnson
Behavioral System Model
in Nursing Practice

Anayis K. Derdiarian

The following case study is chosen because the data contain the problem types proposed by the Model; it is used to demonstrate the application of the model to nursing process. The application of the model to the nursing process includes the generation of nursing data, their analysis and interpretation, in terms of nursing diagnosis, intervention, patient outcomes and evaluation. The data represent the patient's care during the first 24 hours following admission.

ASSESSMENT DATA GATHERING

Using the DBSM instrument interview form, two types of subjective data were generated. The "set" related variables or the variables that potentially predict or influence patient's usual behavior and the behavior resulting from illness. The interview probed into the set, behavioral changes, needs, and goals of the patient in relation to each of the 22 categories. When appropriate, family members provided data. The DBSM-O instrument was used to generate the objective data to identify the problems. The set provided the contextual information to help interpret subjective and objective data in terms of the nursing diagnosis. These variables are categorized as demographic and behavioral.

Set Variables Data. The set variables included demographic profile and behavioral profile data. Mr. T., a 58-year-old Navajo Indian, is admitted for medical evaluation and treatment with radiation of his metastatic mandibular cancer. His wife and daughter accompanied him. He has two daughters, a son, and eight grandchildren. He is cachectic, weak, and his face and nose are swollen. His oral mucosa are covered with thick necrotic exudate, gums are swollen and bleeding, all due to recent chemotherapy, and his breath is foul-smelling. His major complaint is pain in the mouth, inability to chew and swallow, and distress about hospitalization.

The relevant behavioral set data are the following. Achievement: self-sufficient controlling of self, situation, and environment. Affiliation: the head of the family, a family man, a good husband, father, and grandfather, and a committed Christian, active in his church. Aggressive/Protective: protective of self, loved ones, and possessions, and a good provider of financial, psychological, and emotional support. Dependence: does not like to be dependent, he is his own person. Ingestive: enjoys food, especially eating with his family, drinks wine or beer occasionally. Eliminative: no irregularities in bowel movements and urination, and no discharges. Perspires more than his usual, especially at night. Sexual: good marital relationship. Restorative: six-to-seven hours of sleep at night, with interruptions; he takes naps during the day. For relaxation, he used to fish, walk, and visit friends.

Behavioral Change and Patient Goals Data. The DBSM's 22 category interview generated data pertaining to the major changes as a result of illness as well as the positive or negative impact of these changes. The patient ranked the relative importance of these changes on a scale of 1 to 100 (least to most important). Also identified were the factors that are causal or associated with the changes. Next, the patient identified his goals regarding these changes. At the end of each SS data, the patient identified the most important change. Finally, at the end of the SSs' review, the patient was asked to identify the most important change/goal of all the other important changes/goals and rank it. For the intent of this paper, only the data regarding "the most important change" are being re-processed in terms of care plan, as shown in Table 20.1. These change category data are identified by an asterisk. However, data regarding other category changes are provided, as appropriate. Patient goals related to most important changes are identified in the data process outline which follows on page 289.

Table 20.1   Subjective and Objective Behavior Change Data for Assessment by Subsystem and Category

SUBSYSTEM/ CATEGORY	SUBJECTIVE BEHAVIOR DATA	OBJECTIVE DATA
Achievement Category 1.	Decreased/Negative	
*Ability to achieve goals	- Self care and daily living activities due to fatigue and pain	- Self care minimal
		- Does not complete own care, including mouth care
Category 3.		
*Spiritual strength/ hope to achieve through God's help	- Losing hope for healing, this may not be God's will	- Refuses help with mouth care
		- Refuses radiation treatment
Most important change/goal score 85%		
Affiliative Category 2.	Decreased/Negative	
*Belonging or relating to family	- Spending time with family due to poor prognosis	- Withdrawn
		- Interaction with family minimal
	- Eating with family due to his embarrassment related to his inability to chew and without dropping food/fluids from mouth	- Drops food/fluid from mouth
		- Unable to swallow
		- Gags while swallowing
		- Cries insisting to go home
	- Family wants him to be treated sufficiently to enable his care at home. Treatment is not helping. He wants to die at home	
Most important change/goal score 95%.		

Table 20.1   Continued

SUBSYSTEM/ CATEGORY	SUBJECTIVE BEHAVIOR DATA	OBJECTIVE DATA
Aggressive/ Protective Category 2.	Decreased/Negative	
Cognitive reserve or stamina to protect self/ others	- Control over self and situation - Ability to problem-solve	- Cries due to pain but does not request pain medication - Refuses medical treatment - Refuses nursing care
Category 3.		
*Emotional reserve/ Stamina to maintain emotional strength	- Ability to control emotional swings of hopelessness, depression. Not afraid of dying	

Most important change/goal score 90%

Ingestive Category 3.	Decreased/Negative	
*Psychosocial factors affecting eating/drinking for nourishment	- Intake of food/fluids - Eating with family due to mouth condition - Eating native foods due to complications of chemotherapy	- Refuses mouth care to stimulate appetite - Refuses supplemental nourishment - Daily calorie intake is 600 cal. per 24 hours

Most important change/goal 90%. Most important of all the changes/goals: "Being with family as much as possible in the remaining days of his life"; importance score relative to other most important changes/goals 95% (Affiliative SS).

The review of the remaining SSs revealed no significant problems.

Analysis and Interpretation of Data in Terms of Care Plan

The subjective and objective data indicating an actual or potential problem in a SS are analyzed within the parameters of the substructure's set, drive, goal, choice, and action defined in that subsystem. The appropriateness of the behavior or action taken is evaluated in relation to the SS drive and goal and within the context of patient's set, drive, goal, and choice. First, the appropriateness of the patient's goal is evaluated in relation to the SS goal. Next, a general assessment is made to determine the general nature or type of the problem, e.g., insufficient, dominant, discrepant, or incompatible. Third, the appropriateness of the behavior is evaluated in relation to the set variables, choice(s) of behaviors the patient has, and their relation to his goal. Based on the preceding evaluations, a judgment is made as to the appropriateness or effectiveness of the behavior. If inappropriate, the type of problem is determined and a more specific nursing diagnosis is derived and stated. This diagnosis is the foundation of planning the nursing intervention. Each problem in the SS is analyzed using the process discussed previously as the basis for a comprehensive assessment/intervention plan. The "most important" categories are evaluated for priority based on patient's relative importance value as well as the nurse's professional judgment. For the intents of this paper, only the "most important" categories will be analyzed. The preceding analytic process can be learned and it need not be outlined in the detail demonstrated as follows.

Achievement Behavior.   Data analysis and interpretation yielded the following conclusion:

1. Patient's goal: "Gain strength and relief from discomfort." This goal is consistent with the SS's goal and professional judgment.

2. Patient's set: Significant variables include pattern of being in control, ethnicity, gender roles, cancer, poor prognosis, cachexia, and mouth condition.

3. Choice: Of the choices of behaviors available to the patient are to accept help with care, ask for help, accept medical care, and refuse the above.

4. Action: The patient chose the latter.

5. Judgment: The behavior is inadequate to achieve the desired goal, given the set variables of self-sufficiency, able enough to help with own care, controlling self, situation, strong faith in God, and physical/medical conclusion.

6. Type of behavior problem: Insufficiency.

7. Nursing diagnosis: Inadequate assesertiveness in achieving self- , nursing- , and medical-care, all related to weakness and fatigue.

8. Nursing goal/patient outcome: Patient will participate in, accept, and ask for, nursing- and medical-care.

9. Type of nursing intervention indicated: Nurturance, regulation, and stimulation.

10. Specific interventions: Accept patient behavior without judgment (nurturance), counsel patient regarding the relationship between his actions and the desired goal as well as the more appropriate choices, schedule mouth care before meals and sleep and teach him and family member(s) mouth care with gentle techniques. Instruct family to help with mouth care (regulations). Encourage or reinforce improved behavior (Nurturance). Help patient to draw on spiritual strength through his faith and his church (stimulation).

11. Indicators to evaluate patient outcomes: Subjective evidence will include less pain, less fatigue, more comfort. And, objective evidence will include accepting, asking, and participating in self- , nursing- , and medical-care.

Affiliative Behavior.   Data analysis and interpretation yielded the following conclusions:

1. Patient's goal: "To be with family and as much symptom-free as possible, given the poor prognosis." This goal is consistent with the SS and professional judgment.

2. Patient's set: Of significant set variables are roles in family defined by patient's culture, strong family relationships, poor prognosis, and hospitalization.

3. Choice: Of the action alternatives available to him are accept, ask for, participate in, nursing- and medical-care, and leave hospital and refuse care.

4. Action: He chose the latter.

5. Judgment: Patient behavior sufficiently dominant to counteract achieving the desired goal as well as to suppress Achievement and Aggressive/Protective behaviors, given the set variables of strong family relationships, his roles in family, physical/medical condition, and spiritual strength.

6. Type of behavior problem: Dominance.

7. Nursing diagnosis: Strong attachment behavior overpowering the achievement of being and eating with family, related to poor prognosis.

8. Nursing goal/patient outcome: Patient will accept to stay in hospital and comply with nursing- and medical-care.

9. Type of intervention indicated: Nurturance, regulation.

10. Specific interventions: Accept patient behavior without judgment, counsel patient about the relationship of his action to the desired goal as well as the more effective alternative choices. Arrange for physician to counsel patient. Instruct family to discuss with patient their concerns regarding his care at home (regulation). Encourage or reinforce improved behavior.

11. Indicators to evaluate patient outcomes: Subjective evidence will include accepting to stay and receive care, and objective evidence will include cooperating with and participating in nursing- and medical-care.

Aggressive/Protective Behavior. Data analysis and interpretation yielded the following conclusions:

1. Patient's goal: "To recover health and comfort."

2. Patient's set: Of significant set variables are his spiritual strength, family roles as defined by his culture, strong, stable family relationships, cancer, signs and symptoms of disease and its treatment, and poor prognosis.

3.   Choice: Of the behavior alternatives available to him are to seek and/or accept nursing care and medical treatment, problem solve to contend with situations, and be passive about achieving health and comfort.

4.   Action: Patient chose the latter behavior.

5.   Judgment: Behavior discrepant or inconsistent with achieving the desired goal, given the set variables of his spiritual strength, traditional family roles, and physical/medical condition.

6.   Type of behavior problem: Discrepancy.

7.   Nursing Diagnosis: Discrepant or inconsistent behavior to achieve health and comfort related to submissiveness to physical and emotional condition.

8.   Nursing Goal: Patient will assume more control over his situation to preserve and attain health and comfort.

9.   Type of intervention indicated: Nurturance, stimulation, and regulation.

10.   Specific interventions: Accept patient behavior without judgment, counsel patient about the relationship of his behavior to his desired goal as well as the alternative, more appropriate choices. Teach him the importance of appropriate timing of pain medication on its effectiveness. Time and administer the analgesics at regular intervals. Encourage or reinforce improved behavior. Help him to draw strength from his faith.

11.   Indicators to evaluate patient outcomes: Subjective evidence will include acceptance to cooperate with medical treatment and improved pain relief. Objective evidence will include cooperating with medical treatments, accepting or asking for analgesics at appropriate intervals.

Ingestive Behavior Data Analysis and Interpretation Yielded the Following Conclusions:

1.   Patient's goal: "To be able to eat to gain strength to go home and eat with family without embarrassment."

2. Patient's set: Of significant set variables are enjoyment of food, meaning of eating with family as assumed from his culture, tradition of eating with family, condition of mouth, and grossly inadequate caloric/nutritional intake.

3. Choice: Of the significant action alternatives available to the patient are accept mouth care prior to eating to help stimulate appetite, accept supplemental nourishment, ask family to bring ethnic foods permitted by diet restrictions, and refuse/neglect to do the above.

4. Action: Patient chose the latter.

5. Judgment: Action incompatible with the desired goals of the SS as well as those of the Achievement and Affiliative SSs, given his set variables of enjoyment of food and meaning of eating with family, and physical/medical condition.

6. Type of behavior: Incompatibility.

7. Nursing diagnosis: Incompatible behavior to achieve eating to gain strength (Achievement–goal), go home and eat with family without embarrassment (Affiliation–goal).

8. Nursing goal/patient outcome: He will choose to increase intake of nourishment by complying with mouth and diet care; improved laboratory measures.

9. Type of intervention: Nurturance, Regulation, Stimulation, Protection, Control.

10. Specific interventions: Accept behavior without judgment, counsel patient about the relationship of his behavior to his desired goal as well as the more effective alternatives. Help with mouth care before meals. Ask family to bring native foods and encourage/help him eat/drink (protection, stimulation). Encourage or reinforce improved behavior.

11. Indicators to evaluate patient outcomes: Subjective indicators will include increased comfort and appetite. Objective indicators will include increased healing in mouth, reduced foul smell of breath, increased caloric/nutritional intake.

Intra- and Inter-Subsystem Analysis
and Interpretation in Terms of Care Plan

Reviewing the analysis of the intra-SS raw data (Table 20.1), it is pointed out, that the model's use directed and governed the nurse's cognitive processes of analyzing and processing the data. The SS's drive and goals helped 1) to understand the patient's behavior and 2) to evaluate the compatibility, and therefore, the appropriateness, of the patient's drive and goal with the SS's drive and goal. The set variables were used to understand patient's behavior in the context of his own demographic and behavioral profile variables thus, to understand the behavior as being unique to the patient and the situation. Also, set variables were considered in the selection and design of interventions. The choice helped to identify the alternative behaviors or actions available to the patient that could be more effective in meeting his needs. Exploring these with the patient could help to understand the choice of action the patient had taken, or his behavior; it also could help the patient to be aware of other actions. Action helped to identify the behavior in question. Analyzing the behavior in relation to patient's goal, set, and choice, helped to identify its type or nature. This led to specifying the nursing diagnosis. Finally, it is evident that it was the patient's behavior, its effectiveness or ineffectiveness, that was focal to the analysis of the patient's overall, i.e., physical, physiological, psychological/cognitive and emotional, interactive responses to his illness and hospitalization and not just his disease, or singly the signs/symptoms, or psychological, or emotional, responses. Understanding each of the responses is very important, but it is essential to understand how these affect the behavior. It is by manipulating the above that behavior will be modified to be effective to achieve health, comfort, and quality of life. Signs and symptoms, and apparent psychosocial responses will be eliminated or alleviated by focusing on his behavior and its modification. The latter is the nursing focal variable; his disease, signs/symptoms are the interviewing variables and they are the focal variables of the physician. The clear, specific, behavior diagnosis provided the determination of the nursing goal/patient outcome, which, in turn, provided the selection of the appropriate intervention type(s) and the specific interventive modalities. Finally, evaluating the data generated, their interpretation, the diagnosis and the interventions within the SSs are theoretically consistent with the current literature and thus, they are sound.

Reviewing the inter-SS raw data (Table 20.1), it is evident, that the model's proposed interactive and interdependent relationships of the SSs led to the evaluation of SSs' problems in relation to each other. Also, using the model's definition of the Dominance type problem in relation to the definition of the other types, combined with the research findings pertaining to the SSs' interrelationships, led to the identification of the source of the problem.

Analyzing the nature, the relative importance values of the problems, and the relationships among the problems in the SSs, the problem in the Affiliation SS stands out. First, it is the most important change/goal of the patient. Second, it is the most problematic in terms of its interference with his hospitalization and nursing/medical care. Third, because the problem is a dominant type, it is suppressing the Achievement and Aggressive/Protective behaviors. However, this problem is not the first to manage, because it is not the originating change or imbalance in the behavioral system. Its own cause or originating imbalance is rooted in the cognitive aggressive/protective change. He perceives his condition as hopeless, as his poor prognosis limits his chances for survival. Therefore, he wishes to be with family and die at home. Thus, it is most plausible that while the overall intervention is multi-system, the initial intervention concentrates on the prescriptions for an Aggressive/Protective Category 2 problem. By implementing these interventions, the cognitive set of the patient could be managed to restore cognitive protective abilities, control, and balance. If the latter outcomes are achieved, the patient would resume control of self, situation, environment and thus, be more likely to participate in his care to achieve self-care, comfort, relief from pain, increased intake of food and consequently strength. It is evident that by intervening in the Aggressive/Protective SS, the interventions would also be effective in indirectly intervening in the problems in the Achievement and Ingestive SSs, and, ultimately, in the Affiliative SS problem. It is also evident, that interventions in the Aggressive/Protective SS problem will have potentiating effect on the interventions prescribed for the problems in the Affiliative, Achievement, and Ingestive SSs.

The preceding discussion in relation to problem ranking is theoretically sound. As demonstrated in earlier studies, changes in the Aggressive/Protective SS are directly and also indirectly related to the Achievement, Affiliative, and Ingestive SS changes. Therefore, extrapolating that intervening in Aggressive/Protective SS could directly and also indirectly achieve balance in all of the affected SSs is also theoretically sound. It is evident that the above analysis would make patient's problem management, as directed by the theory, more rational and thus, more effective and economical.

CONCLUSIONS

Concluding the preceding analysis, it is clear that the model provided a comprehensive scope for assessing and intervening in the patient's multiple problems. It also provided a focus in pointing to the patient's behavior as being central to nursing's understanding and action. It provided an understanding of the nature of patient problems expressed in the types of those problems. It provided awareness of the nature of nursing action, role, and intervention in relation to the patient's problem. Finally, it provided a perspective and a context unique to nursing, but congruent with the contexts of other professions' actions. It did this by providing a view of the patient, a view of patient problems central to nursing management, and a view of nursing's action, thus clarifying the nursing's view of the patient as being from, but in relation to, the views of other related professions. In its perspective it provided the foundations for nursing's theoretical, methodological, and practice development.

Implications for Generalizability of JBS Model in Nursing Practice

In its current state of specification, the model has immediate and future applicability to practice. The model's immediate generalizability has been tested on adult patients with cancer, myocardial infarct (MI) treated either medically or surgically, patients with specific cancers, and patients with AIDS. In the future, the model's already developed theoretical constructs could be operationally defined to suit other patient populations defined by age, gender, medical diagnosis, medical treatment, or other appropriate characteristics. The theoretical constructs, the instruments, the data generated, and the methodology of specification of a model can be taught in schools and continuing education as a basis for practice. Thus, they can advance practice, education, and research in nursing, within the realm of nursing defined by this model. The relationship of the model to the above is outlined in Figure 20.1.

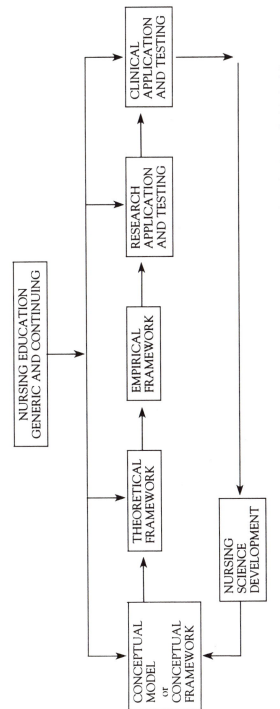

Figure 20.1 The relationship of nursing models and nursing research, practice, and education based on the Scientific Method Process.

The evolution of this model's development and testing demonstrates its scientific and clinical background. As such, it compels nursing's serious efforts to endorse this model in its educational, practice, and research endeavors. Further scientific testing of this model is warranted in two equally essential and interactive methods—Research and Clinical. Areas for testing could be focused on the SSs individually or collectively, Nursing Diagnoses and their typology within and among the SS. The relationships of set, drive, action, choice, and goal to SS behavior could be studied. The relationships among the SSs could be studied. And, finally, the relationship of the intervention typologies and the nursing problem typologies could be studied.

Appendix I

Resources for Nursing

Appendix 1

Resources for Nursing Theories in Practice

Cathie L. Wallace

This appendix provides sources for readers seeking additional information for study and use of the major nursing theories presented in *Nursing Theories in Practice* (Parker, 1990) and this book. Each nursing theorist who contributed to these two volumes was invited to submit descriptions of organizations or associations of nurses which support and contribute to development and use of their theory. Their responses are combined with other published sources to provide a composite listing of key references for nurses desiring to connect with others using specific nursing theories in practice.

Sources for a theory include one or more of the following: descriptions of organizations or associations supportive of the nursing theory; official journal, newsletter, or other publication of the organization or association; organizations or individual nurses applying specific theories in practice or in a practice setting. This compilation of important sources is not meant to be exhaustive, but will give readers a place to begin their personal search for like-minded colleagues. You are referred to the nursing periodical literature for the most current applications for each major nursing theory.

Theorists are listed alphabetically in the pages to follow. Addresses and telephone numbers for resources are given, where possible, to facilitate the reader's explorations. One association concerned with nursing theory of interest to several theorists can be found at the end of the appendix.

ANNE BOYKIN & SAVINA O. SCHOENHOFER

Please see Savina O. Schoenhofer and Anne Boykin on page 309.

MADELEINE LEININGER

Dr. Leininger founded the Transcultural Nursing Society (TCNS) in 1974 as a worldwide organization for nurses interested in and prepared to advance transcultural nursing. The Transcultural Nursing Society serves as a forum to bring nurses together from around the world with common and diverse interests to improve care to culturally diverse people.

The *Journal of Transcultural Nursing*, the official journal of the Transcultural Nursing Society, was created in 1989 to advance transcultural nursing knowledge and practices by providing substantive content which focuses on transcultural nursing theory, research and practice. A subscription to this semi-annual, juried publication and other current educational and service resources of the Society are included in TCNS membership dues.

For further information about transcultural nursing contact:

Transcultural Nursing Society
Madonna College
Division of Nursing & Health
36600 Schoolcraft Road
Livonia, MI 48150-1173
Phone: (313) 592-5155

Executive Coordinator:
Peggy Shinkel

Secretary:
Donna Barnes

For information about the *Journal of Transcultural Nursing* contact:

Journal of Transcultural Nursing
University of Tennessee, Memphis
College of Nursing
Continuing Education
877 Madison Avenue
Memphis, TN 38163

Dr. Leininger also founded the International Association for Human Caring, which is fully described later in this appendix.

MYRA E. LEVINE

To obtain further information regarding the use of Levine's Conservation Model in practice contact:

Myra E. Levine, MSN, RN, FAAN
Professor Emerita
College of Nursing
University of Illinois at Chicago
Chicago, Illinois

or

Jane Pond, MSN, RNC, CRNP
Nursing Director, Homeless Programs
Philadelphia Health Management Corporation
Philadelphia, Pennsylvania

or

Karen Moore Schaefer, DNSc, RN
Associate Professor
Allentown College of St. Francis de Sales
Center Valley, Pennsylvania
Nurse Researcher
The Allentown Hospital-Lehigh Valley Hospital Center
Allentown, Pennsylvania

BETTY NEUMAN

The Neuman Systems Model Trustees Group was established in the fall of 1988 to preserve, protect, and perpetuate the integrity of the Neuman Systems Model for the future of nursing. Anyone interested in the use, continuing development and evaluation of the model may become associate members. International Neuman System Model Symposiums are held biennially. Archives containing historical information about the Neuman Systems Model and Dr. Neuman's papers and writings are housed at Neumann College, Aston, Pennsylvania.

For information about the Trustees Group contact:

The Neuman Systems Model Trustees Group, Inc.
P.O. Box 488
Beverly, OH 45715

For information regarding membership contact:

Dr. Lois W. Lowry, DNSc, RN
Assistant Professor
University of South Florida, College of Nursing
Health Sciences Center, Box 22
12901 Bruce B. Downs
Tampa, FL 33612-4799
Phone: (813) 972-4011
Fax: (813) 974-5418

Neuman News is a newsletter published annually by the Neuman Systems Model Trustee Group to keep the nursing community informed about the development and use of the Neuman Systems Model, to enhance networking among Neuman Model users, and to keep users informed of current research, publications, and symposia related to the model.

Neuman News Editor:

Dr. Cynthia Flynn Capers, PhD, RN
Associate Professor
Thomas Jefferson University
College of Allied Health Sciences
Nursing Department, Office 1251
130 S. 9th St.
Philadelphia, PA 19107

MARGARET NEWMAN

The Healing Web, a collaboration among Augustana College, Sioux Valley Hospital, and the University of South Dakota, uses Newman's Theory of Health as a basis for practice and education. Readers interested in the use of Newman's theory in practice may contact Healing Web member:

JoEllen Koerner
Vice President of Patient Services
Sioux Valley Hospital
1100 South Euclid Ave.
PO Box 5039
Sioux Falls, SD 57117-5039
Phone: (605) 333-1000

Nurses interested in the congruence of Newman's theory with nurse case management practice may contact:

Gerri Lamb, PhD, RN
Cathy Michaels, PhD, RN
Directors of Clinical Research and
Nurse Case Managers
Carondelet St. Mary's Hospital and Health Center
1601 West St. Mary's Road
Tucson, AZ 85745
Phone: (602) 622-5833

DOROTHEA E. OREM

The International Orem Society for Nursing Science and Scholarship was founded to advance nursing science and scholarship through the use of Dorothea E. Orem's nursing conceptualizations in nursing education, practice, and research. Annual Self-Care Deficit Nursing Theory (S-CDNT) institutes examine theoretical concepts and practical applications of Self-Care Deficit Nursing Theory, and a series of International Conferences has been initiated.

For information about individual or organizational membership contact:

Marjorie Isenberg, DNSc, RN, FAAN
Wayne State University
College of Nursing
5557 Cass Avenue, Room 368
Detroit, MI 48202

or

Susan Taylor, PhD, RN, FAAN
S428 School of Nursing

University of Missouri-Columbia
Columbia, MO 65211

The *Self-Care Deficit Nursing Theory Newsletter* is now the publication of the International Orem Society. Submissions related to nursing research, applications of S-CDNT in practice and education, applications in private practice or in health care agencies and institutions should be sent to:

Self-Care Deficit Nursing Theory Newsletter
c/o Dr. Susan Taylor, Co-Chair
International Orem Society Publications Committee
School of Nursing
University of Missouri-Columbia
Columbia, MO 65211

ROSEMARIE RIZZO PARSE

The goal of the International Consortium of Parse Scholars is to foster excellence in nursing through theory development, research, and practice with Parse's theory of human becoming. The Consortium holds annual Fall Weekend Seminars with scholarly presentations and publishes *Illuminations*. Nurses interested in pursuing the goal of the organization may contact:

Gail J. Mitchell, PhD, RN, President
International Consortium of Parse Scholars
Ste. 1311-99 Harbour Square
Toronto, Ontario, Canada M5J 2H2
Phone: (416) 603-8522

JOSEPHINE PATERSON & LORETTA ZDERAD

Nurses interested in the application of Humanistic Nursing Theory in the primary health care context may contact:

Nancy O'Connor, MSN, RN
Assistant Professor of Nursing
Oakland University
Rochester, MI 48309-4401
Phone: (313) 370-4076

Readers engaging in specialty practice and acute and long-term care settings make contact:

Dr. Doris Hines
Rural Route #1, Box 341
Agency, MO 64401
Phone: (816) 253-9443

MARTHA E. ROGERS

The Society of Rogerian Scholars (SRS) is a formal, organized structure for the stimulation, development, and exchange of ideas related to Rogerian Science of Unitary Human Beings. The Mission of the Society is to advance nursing as a science through an emphasis on the Science of Unitary Human Beings and to contribute significantly to the knowledgeable nursing of human beings. The focus of the Society is education, research, and practice in service of humankind.

The Society of Rogerian Scholars has eight regions, with several offering regional Rogerian conferences twice per year. *Rogerian Nursing Science News: The Newsletter of the Society of Rogerian Scholars* is published quarterly. The new official journal of the SRS, *Visions: The Journal of Rogerian Nursing Science*, is an annual publication.

For information about membership contact:

The Society of Rogerian Scholars, Inc.
437 Twin Bay Drive
Pensacola, FL 32534
Phone: (904) 474-9793
Contact person: Sheila Morrisey

SISTER CALLISTA ROY

Readers interested in studying and using the Roy Adaptation Model may contact:

Sister Callista Roy, PhD, RN, FAAN
Professor of Nursing
Boston College
Chestnut Hill, Massachusetts

Research Professor in Nursing
Mount St. Mary's College
Los Angeles, California

or

Boston-Based Adaptation Research in Nursing Society (BBARNS)

Purposes:

- to advance nursing practice by developing basic and clinical nursing knowledge based on the model.

- to provide the scholarly colleagueship needed for knowledge development and research.

- to enhance networks of dissemination of research for practice.

- to encourage scholars in the field and facilitate related programs of research.

Core Group meets quarterly and shares scholarly and organizational responsibilities.

Key Contact:

Mary E. Duffy, PhD, RN
Professor and Director
Center for Nursing
Attn: BBARNS Core Group
211 Cushing Hall
Boston College School of Nursing
Chestnut Hill, MA 02167
Phone: (617) 552-3123
FAX: (617) 552-0745

Sr. Callista Roy Annual Lectureship and Conference

Purposes:

- to recognize the leadership role of Mount St. Mary's College Department of Nursing, chaired by Dr. Roy, in the initial development of the Roy Adaptation Model.

- to address contemporary issues in practice and education from the perspective of the model.

Conferences held each Fall at:

Mount St. Mary's College
Department of Nursing
12001 Chalon Road
Los Angeles, CA 90049
Phone: (310) 476-2237

SAVINA O. SCHOENHOFER and ANNE BOYKIN

Nurses interested in applying the theory of Nursing as Caring in their practice may contact:

Anne Boykin, PhD, RN
Dean, College of Nursing
Florida Atlantic University
500 NW 20th Street
Boca Raton, FL 33431
Phone: (407) 367-3260
Fax: (407) 367-3687

   or

Savina Schoenhofer, PhD, RN
Associate Professor
Graduate Program Director
College of Nursing
500 NW 20th Street
Boca Raton, FL 33431
Phone: (407) 367-3260
Fax: (407) 367-3687

JEAN WATSON

Readers seeking to connect with nurses who apply Watson's theory of human caring as a clinical practice model may contact:

Eileen Cappell, Project Development Nurse
Baycrest Centre for Geriatric Care
3560 Bathurst Street
North York, Ontario M6A 2El CANADA
Phone: (416) 789-5131 Extension 2118

   or

Ruth Neil, PhD, RN
Project Director, The Caring Center
Denver Nursing Project in Human Caring
VAMC, Building 5
1055 Clermont Street
Denver, CO 80220
Phone: (303) 393-4616

> or

Jean Watson, PhD, RN, FAAN, Project Director, Fuld ND grant
Sally Phillips, PhD, RN, Director
Nursing Doctorate (ND) Program
Pilot program in human caring, health and healing
University of Colorado School of Nursing
4200 East Ninth Avenue, Box C288
Denver, CO 80262

LORETTA ZDERAD and JOSEPHINE PATERSON

Please see Josephine Paterson and Loretta Zderad on page 306.

Other Associations Which Support Nurses Interested in the Study and Use of Nursing Theory in Practice

INTERNATIONAL ASSOCIATION FOR HUMAN CARING

The International Association for Human Caring (IAHC) serves as a scholarly forum for nurses to advance knowledge of care and caring within the discipline of nursing. This association may be a useful resource for nurses using several of the major nursing theories described in *Nursing Theories in Practice* (Parker, 1990) and this book.

For information regarding membership in IAHC contact:

International Association for Human Caring
Business Office
Division of Nursing
3900 University Blvd.
Tyler, TX 75701-6699

All members of the IAHC receive the *International Association for Human Caring Newsletter* which is published bi-yearly Fall and Spring. IAHC members may submit materials for the newsletter to:

International Association for Human Caring Newsletter
UTHSC at Houston School of Nursing
1100 Holcombe Blvd., 5th Floor
Houston, TX 77030